The Reflux Book is a wonde̲ ̲̲̲̲̲̲̲̲̲̲̲̲̲̲̲̲-
cians. The information is presented in a simple, clear manner that
will not intimidate parents. And, it is extremely thorough and accurate which will appeal to clinicians working with children who are
dealing with reflux. Every therapist working with children who
have a feeding difficulty should have one!
*Krisi Brackett MS CCC-SLP, The Pediatric Feeding and Dysphagia
Newsletter*

◆

A smart, concise, and supportive resource for concerned parents of
children with reflux. The author's years of experience facilitating
parent support groups, publishing, and navigating her own children's health care needs, have provided her with a great deal of
common sense and practical advice. Anderson clearly connects with
her readers, and her readers will connect with her.
*Hope Trachtenberg-Fifer RN, MS. Certified Health Education Special-
ist, Member, American Medical Writers Association*

◆

The book is very thorough, It contains a lot of complex scientific
information expressed very simply.
Vik Khoshoo, MD, PhD, Pediatric Gastroenterologist

◆

If you are a parent with young children, you must read this book.
Rick M, Alpharetta, GA, Parent of a child with reflux

◆

The Reflux Book is a must for all parents of children suffering with
gastroesophageal reflux disease (GERD).

Section 1 of the book is a basic overview. The book starts out with
an excellent introduction to acid reflux. In Chapter 1, normal digestion is discussed, and then reflux is defined. Reflux is compared to
colic, and parents are reassured that reflux is very common. Chapters 2 and 3 give a great description of symptoms your child may be
experiencing, and clues that should prompt a trip to see the child's
physician. You will again be reassured to know how common acid

reflux is, and how your child's doctor might go about making the proper diagnosis.

Treating Infant Reflux: Chapters 4 through 9 go over the treatment of gastroesophageal reflux disease in children including preparing your home to best care for your child with GERD andfeeding tips, including how often and what to feed your child. These measures are reviewed in detail. Then various medications used to treat GERD in children is discussed.

Throughout the book, the general theme is to provide an informative resource for parents of children afflicted with this disease, while doing so in a non-threatening way. While many medical books for the layperson tend to scare those that read it with the attitude of an alarmist, The Reflux Book has a straight-forward and positive approach. It should be read by all who are close to a child with gastroesophageal reflux disease.

Todd Eisner, MD, Gastroenterologist and writer for HealthCentral.com

The Reflux Book

This book belongs to:

The Reflux Book

By

Beth Pulsifer-Anderson

Foreword by Bill Sears, MD

The Reflux Book
Copyright © 2007 Beth Pulsifer-Anderson

Disclaimer: This book is not a substitute for medical care and advice. Please consult your physician before starting, modifying or discontinuing any medication or treatment. This book is not a publication of the Pediatric Adolescent Gastroesophageal Reflux Association (PAGER)

All Illustrations © The Reflux Book 2007
Illustrations 1, 2, 3, 4 drawn by Megan Clayton
Illustrations 5, 6, 7, 8 drawn by Kristen A. Davis
Illustration 9 drawn by Chris Anderson
Front Cover Photo © 2007 Carolyn Sandstrom
Welcome to Holland © 1987 Emily Perl Kingsley with permission

I would love to hear from you. Send inquires, corrections, additions comments and stories to:
Intensive Care Parenting, LLC
Beth Anderson
PO Box 454
Garrett Park, MD 20896
www.refluxbook.com
author@refluxbook.com

This book was self-published and may undergo many small changes over time. The book you are holding was printed in August 2008.

Library binding and quantity discounts are available. Details can be found at www.refluxbook.com

616.3 Medical – Diseases - Digestive

This book is dedicated to:

Katie, Chris and Eric

TABLE OF CONTENTS

SECTION 2 - ADVANCED CONCEPTS

THANKS

I am eternally grateful to the hundreds of volunteers and families who shared their stories with me over the past fifteen years. Your stories are wonderful and add so much to this book.

I would like to thank the Pediatric Adolescent Gasroesophageal Reflux Association Board of Directors for their ongoing support. Thanks to Sara Hunt and Tracey Butler for gathering material and organizing earlier material. A special thanks to Caroline McGraw and her amazing family for their contribution to the organization in the early years. A million thanks to Jan Gambino for her hard work on another project focused on GERD which we co-authored and which serves as the basis for this book. Thanks to Hank Abromson for all the help when this project got bogged down.

Thanks to Dr. Sears for encouragement and guidance during the book writing process. I have admired Dr. Bill's work for years - he was the first to write about reflux in his parenting books. Thank you to Megan Clayton and Kristin Davis for creating the illustration in the book. And thank you to Emily Perl Kingsley for allowing us to reprint her essay, Welcome to Holland. Thank you to Carolyn Sandstrom for taking the touching photo on the cover. Thanks to Danielle Porter for all her help with publicity.

Thank you to the many people who gave feedback: Joel Campbell, PhD, Mary Biden Bourgeois, Stephanie Doersam, Pam Tyler, Amy Arnold, Stephanie Petters, Jacque Pulsifer, Al Reynolds and Vic Khoshoo, MD. They caught most of my mistakes - any that remain are purely mine.

I also want to thank my wonderful husband, Eric, for taking on more than his share of the house and financial burden for the last fifteen years when the reflux families needed my help. My parents, Jacque and Al Pulsifer deserve a huge thanks for all their help keeping the house and family together during the worst reflux years and the book writing months. I would like to thank Leah Brasch, MD for going beyond the call of duty when caring for Katie. My friends, Jacqueline Barth, Lisa Tragert, Bernadette Knoebel and Sue Hosford saved my sanity when the kids were little and remained close after the crisis years. (Jacqueline is the neighbor featured in one of the vignettes who took my kids when I just couldn't take another second listening to Katie cry.) I would like to thank Sharon Tiano who ran a small reflux support group in Boston – she was my mentor in starting a support group.

Above all, I would also like to thank Katie and Chris for allowing their stories to be shared in this book and for all the on-the-job-training you guys gave me. I love you.

FOREWORD

This book is a must-read for any family who has an infant or child with gastroesophageal reflux (GER).

My interest in GER began in the early nineties when, as a pediatrician, I was uncomfortable passing babies off as having "colic." I still remember a mother coming into my office with her one-month-old baby who sounded like she had typical "colic." The mother said to me, "Dr. Bill, I know my baby is hurting somewhere and I'm going to camp out in your office until you find out why she is hurting." This mother encouraged me to keep searching for why her baby hurt, and the cause of the "colic" turned out to be severe gastroesophageal reflux.

Since that time, I have replaced the term "colicky baby" with the more accurate description "the hurting baby," and it turns out that many so-called colicky babies actually suffer from this treatable condition.

GER is tough on the child and the family. Hurting babies, sleepless nights, tired parents – that's what happens in a reflux family. The information in this book has been compiled by authors and parents who have survived and thrived with their infants and children with reflux and have shared their wisdom to help other parents who have children with this condition.

My favorite feature of this book is that it teaches what I believe is the best medical model for the treatment of GER: the pills-and-skills model. This is the model that I follow in my pediatric practice in treating infants and children with GER. Besides the "pills," or medications, that you will learn about to treat GER, you will also learn the many infant and childcare skills and feeding skills that will help alleviate this painful

iii

condition. For example, in my office the first skill I give parents is what my patients dub Dr. Bill's rule of reflux: "Feed your baby half as much, twice as often." For the older child I add, "…and chew twice as long." For the younger baby we often add the next rule, "Keep baby upright and quiet for 20-30 minutes after a feeding." These are just a couple of the home remedies for reflux that you will learn about throughout this book. I wish that every healthcare provider who counsels parents for GER will "prescribe" this book.

William Sears, M.D.

Co-author, THE BABY BOOK

Dr. Bill is an Associate Clinical Professor of Pediatrics at the University of California, Irvine, School of Medicine. Dr. Bill received his pediatric training at Harvard Medical School's Children's Hospital in Boston and The Hospital for Sick Children in Toronto -- the largest children's hospital in the world, where he served as associate ward chief of the newborn nursery and associate professor of pediatrics. Dr. Sears is a fellow of the American Academy of Pediatrics (AAP) and a fellow of the Royal College of Pediatricians (RCP). Dr. Bill is also a medical and parenting consultant for BabyTalk and Parenting magazines and the pediatrician on the website Parenting.com. Dr. Sears is the author or co-author of 30+ books on parenting and children's health.

HOW TO USE THIS BOOK

Hello, and welcome to the world of acid reflux. The book is a comprehensive handbook for families and caregivers of children with gastroesophageal reflux and related disorders. I hope I can guide you in your search for answers and offer some support and comfort during a stressful time in your life.

Remember that the information in this book is not a substitute for medical advice. A physician or other medical professional needs to be consulted to make an accurate diagnosis and provide a treatment plan. You should not try any treatment, positioning or medication without first discussing the topic with your doctor.

Keep in mind that some of the treatments and trends presented in this book will be replaced with new and better ideas as medicine changes rapidly. The treatments for pediatric reflux have changed significantly even in the past 17 years since my own little refluxers were babies! The Pediatric Adolescent Gastroesophageal Reflux Association website at www.reflux.org is a good place to search for information on the latest in research and treatment. And most importantly of all, consult with your child's doctor for information on the best treatment approach.

Which Parts of this Book Should You Read?

I hope that you will find this book both interesting and valuable. I realize that many of you will have to hire a live-in baby sitter in order to get the time to read it! Since it might be unrealistic, and probably unnecessary to read the whole book, I have provided a detailed Table of Contents. This will allow you to choose the section you need most today.

I suggest that everybody start by reading the basic chapters. If your child spits up a lot but is not experiencing medical problems, the first chapters will be helpful, but the later chapters will just be scary and overwhelming. If your child has mild symptoms but they aren't causing big problems, you may want to read a few more chapters. Those of you with babies and toddlers who have many symptoms may need to read more. If you have older children, you may want to read more of the chapters toward the back of the book.

Most of the book focuses on infants and toddlers with reflux. I have provided information on older children and children with complex medical issues related to reflux in the Advanced Section. If you have a baby with typical reflux symptoms, you will save yourself a lot of worry by skipping the Advanced Section. You might want to read the table of contents closely – then if your child starts to develop problems such as food aversion, you will know there is a chapter you can read later.

Parents of children with reflux sometimes call their babies "refluxers" or "gerdlings." It isn't very politically correct to call a baby by their medical condition, but parents like to use the term because it seems more cute than clinical. You will see it in some of the stories.

I use the pronoun "she" throughout the book because my worst refluxer was a girl!

There are many references in the book to the Pediatric Adolescent Gastroesophageal Reflux Association - PAGER Association for short. I am the founder and Executive Director of PAGER Association. The organization was originally formed in 1992 as a local support group in suburban Maryland. Since then, the organization has grown to be a large, well-regarded non-profit patient support organization with a busy website, a quarterly newsletter and parent friendly medical information. Trained parent volunteers provide one-to-one support to parents via phone and email.

Throughout the book are many personal stories and vignettes in italics. The families you will meet in this book are real, but some of the details of their stories have blurred over the years. After talking to hundreds of parents, I can no longer remember many of the names that go with the stories. If you recognize yourself in one of these stories it may be a coincidence, or you may be an old friend and I would love to hear from you again. Please send updates and more vignettes.

Nobody volunteers to come to the world of reflux. It can be confusing and stressful. I hope this book will help you on your journey. Perhaps it will even help some of you to find your way home. I hope that the voices of other parents will offer you company and hope along this often-bumpy road.

Most of what I learned about acid reflux was through on-the-job training - from living with my gerdlings day in and day out. What my kids didn't teach me about acid reflux, I learned through hundreds of calls and e-mails from parents and other caregivers from around the world who have contacted the Pediatric Adolescent Gastroesophageal Reflux Association for support and information. I also read hundreds of medical journal articles on reflux and attended many medical conferences.

It was very difficult to decide how much information to include in this book. I received a lot of suggestions and help from various reviewers, but ultimately, the decision about what to include was mine. I believe that parents are entitled to full information, but at the same time, I don't want to scare readers. This was a very tough balancing act and I probably didn't fully succeed. Even the cover of the book sparked lively discussions - several doctors thought it was too depressing but parents loved it.

I hope that this book will help both you and your child. Life with reflux is very stressful, but you are not alone.

Beth Anderson

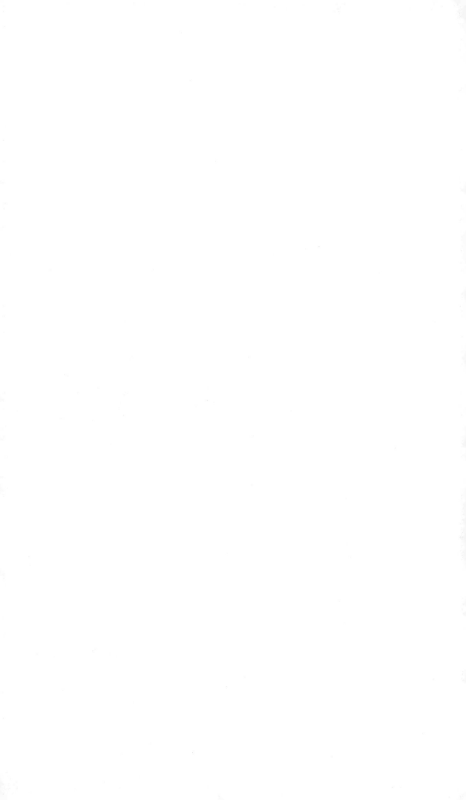

Welcome to Holland

By Emily Perl Kingsley

I am often asked to describe the experience of raising a child with a disability - to try to help people who have not shared that unique experience to understand it, to imagine how it would feel.

It's like this . . . When you're going to have a baby; it's like planning a fabulous vacation trip - to Italy. You buy a bunch of guidebooks and make your wonderful plans. The Coliseum, the Michelangelo David, the gondolas in Venice. You may learn some handy phrases in Italian. It's all very exciting. After months of eager anticipation, the day finally arrives. You pack your bags and off you go. Several hours later, the plane lands. The stewardess comes and says, "Welcome to Holland." "Holland?" you say. "What do you mean Holland? I signed up for Italy! I'm supposed to be in Italy. All my life I've dreamed of going to Italy." But there's been a change in the flight plan. They've landed in Holland and there you must stay.

The important thing is that they haven't taken you to a horrible, disgusting, filthy place full of pestilence, famine and disease. It's just a different place. So you go out and buy new guidebooks. And you must learn a whole new language. And you will meet a whole new group of people you would never have met. It's just a different place. It's slower paced than Italy, less flashy than Italy. But after you've been there for a while and you catch your breath, you look around, and you begin to notice that Holland has windmills, Holland has tulips, Holland even has Rembrandts. But everyone you know is busy coming and going from Italy, and they're all bragging about what a wonderful time they had there. And for the rest of your life, you will say, "Yes, that's where I was supposed to go. That's what I had planned." The pain of that will never go away, because the loss of that dream is a very significant loss. But if you spend your life mourning the fact that you didn't get to Italy, you will never be free to enjoy the very special, very lovely things about Holland.

Reprinted with permission from Emily Perl Kingsley. Her son has special needs and reflux. This is the original version of her essay.

Section 1

Basics

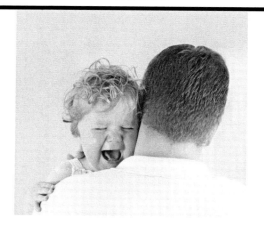

1 ACID REFLUX 101

Many of you sat in high school biology class and thought, "I will never need to know any of this information!" Fast forward to parenthood and maybe now you are wishing you could remember more about the lecture on digestion. For those of you who are too tired to remember your phone number, much less what you learned in high school biology class, this chapter starts with a refresher. So welcome to anatomy class ... again.

Remember, if this chapter still leaves you with questions about the mechanics of reflux, ask your doctor for a quick lesson. All of those colorful charts and pictures in their exam rooms are not just for decoration.

Normal Digestion

When you eat, food is chewed, mixed with saliva and swallowed. It passes to the very back of the pharynx (back of the mouth). The food passes behind the trachea (windpipe) which gets covered by a flap of muscle called the epiglottis.

The swallowed food passes a ring of muscles high in the esophagus (Upper Esophageal Sphincter /UES) that opens to let the food pass and then closes. The esophagus produces mucus to help the food slide down better. The esophageal muscles contract with a wave-like motion to squeeze the food downward past another sphincter (Lower Esophageal Sphincter/LES) and into the stomach. The muscles of your esophagus are so strong you can swallow when you are standing on your head.

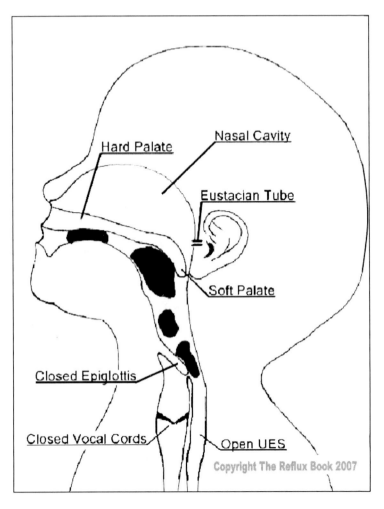

Illustration 1. *Swallowing: The soft palate (soft area toward the back of the roof of the mouth) rises to block off the nasal cavity and Eustachian tubes. The food moves past the closed epiglottis and down the esopha-gus to the stomach. The epiglottis and vocal cords are closed and the Upper Esophageal Sphincter (UES) is open.*

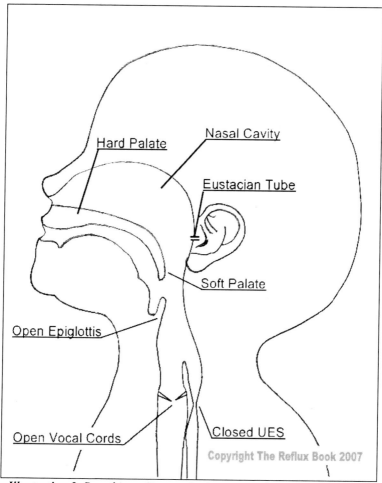

Illustration 2. *Breathing: Air goes in the nose and mouth, through the trachea, past the vocal cords and into the lungs. The epiglottis is open and the Upper Esophageal Sphincter (UES) is closed.*

The stomach stretches slowly to accommodate the food (gastric accommodation) and then signals the body to stop eating when it is full. The stomach muscles start squeezing, grinding and churning the food to break it into smaller parts. Soft foods and liquids trigger milder squeezing and solid foods trigger vigorous churning action.

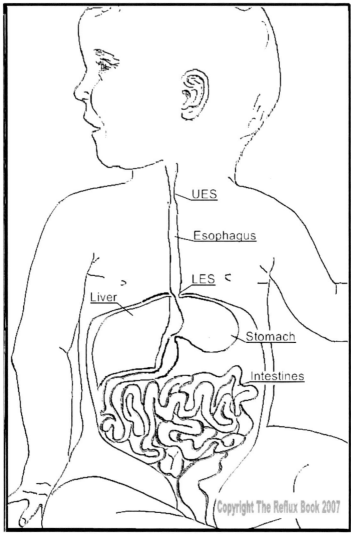

Illustration 3: The Digestive System

The Myth of the Flappy Thingy
The area where the esophagus meets the stomach is called the Lower Esophageal Sphincter and it is a ring of muscles. Many doctors refer to it as a flap because that is easier to visualize.

The walls of the stomach produce acid and enzymes to help break down the food. The stomach lining is made of cells that are not normally damaged by acid.

The stomach grinds the food into mush, and then the food passes through the pyloric sphincter/valve at the bottom of the stomach and into the duodenum, which is the top portion of the small intestine. The time this takes varies greatly from person to person and from meal to meal. Fatty foods and tough foods like meat and seeds stay in the stomach longer than mushy foods or liquids.

When the food is in the small intestine, it mixes with enzymes, bile and alkaline secretions, which help to break up the food and release the nutrients. The pancreas and the liver make enzymes and bile that are stored in the gall bladder. Most of the nutrients are absorbed through the wall of the small intestine and the waste passes into the large intestine. There the water is removed so the waste gets more solid.

Other components of digestion are the brain, which signals the body to eat, the nose, which stimulates the appetite, teeth for chewing, and saliva glands that wet the food.

Defining "Reflux"

A full description of reflux is 50% medicine and 50% careful wording.

The simplest definition of reflux is backwashing of stomach contents into the esophagus. It is literally that simple.

Gastro	+	Esophageal	+	Reflux
(Stomach)		(Throat)		(Backwash)

But, the word *reflux* is a lot like the word *depression*. It is commonly used to describe something that can range from trivial and annoying to something that is very serious indeed. When somebody says they are depressed, they might be telling you they are upset over a temporary situation or they might be telling you that they have been hospitalized. The word depression covers a very broad spectrum. So does the word reflux.

The real problem in describing reflux is that there are a million levels of reflux ranging from normal to life threatening. Somehow, I had to take those million variations and group them into useful categories. At the same time, I have to explain what reflux ISN'T.

PLEASE, don't get too hung up on the way I divided reflux into three categories. They are not set in stone and they are not the only way to divide reflux.

When I was asking doctors to help me come up with a definition, they all gave definitions that contradicted each other in subtle ways. And every attempt at revision provoked new discussions.

Some reviewers were 'lumpers' and wanted to divide reflux into two categories (disease and not disease). Others were 'splitters' who like more categories. Some call normal spit up 'Gastroesophageal Reflux' and some said, 'Don't use a medical sounding term for something that is normal.' Some doctors advised using clinical terms throughout the book and others advised using a more conversational tone and only using clinical terms occasionally. Some suggested giving you a list of every term you will see if you read medical journals and magazines. Others found the list too confusing or said to move terms to a different category – this is why you will see some overlap in the terminology table.

The categories I use are the best compromise I could come up with. They aren't perfect, but they are reasonably accurate and fairly easy to understand. Ask your doctors what categories they use.

There are many legitimate ways to describe the various levels of reflux. I chose to use these:

Reflux – The Normal Event
Reflux – The Condition/Illness
Reflux – The Disease

Reflux - The Normal Event

The simplest definition of reflux is the backwashing of stomach contents up into the esophagus and occasionally out of the mouth. In fact, the word reflux is just Latin for reverse flow.

But this isn't a disease - it is a normal process that happens to almost everybody after meals. Adults call it a "wet burp" and in babies, wet burps often come up all the way out of the mouth and become known as "spit up."

When babies spit up a lot, the parents often get quite worried even though the doctor will view the spitting as more of a laundry problem than a true medical problem. Rest assured that occasional episodes of reflux are very seldom cause for alarm. Even a bit of spitting up after every meal can be perfectly normal and harmless (at least to the baby). Doctors often refer to this as "physiologic" (normal) reflux.

If your child has this harmless level of reflux, you will not need to read the more technical parts of this book, but you may find that the feeding, diet and positioning ideas can help quite a bit.

The term 'normal reflux' or 'reflux events' will be used in this book when it is necessary to distinguish it from other levels of reflux.

Reflux - The Condition or Illness

Most people, including doctors, use the words *condition*, *illness* and *disease* to mean the same thing, but they aren't quite the same.

The medical definition of a *condition* is an excessive amount of what healthy bodies normally do. In this case, we are talking about an unusually large number of reflux episodes. A child who experiences an excessive number of reflux episodes may require a lot of extra work, but this is really a condition, not a disease. (Disease is covered in the next section.)

In medical lingo, an *illness* is when the patient or their family quite rightly believes there is a problem but it isn't serious enough for the doctors to call it a *disease*. A child who fusses a lot during feeding may be experiencing reflux that makes her parent know that something is wrong, but the doctor may not think the problem is severe enough to treat with medication.

It is quite natural to be worried when your child is doing something all day long that other children only do occasionally. Excessive reflux events or crying can be quite stressful on parents and the whole family.

The home care and coping strategies in this book may be quite useful for this level of reflux. If your child has this level of reflux, it is also important for you to really understand the condition well enough that you can help monitor your child carefully. Her symptoms will probably get better with time, but if the symptoms get worse, she may get a diagnosis of reflux disease, which is described next. Recognizing problems early can help reduce her suffering.

The term 'reflux the condition' will be used in this book when it is necessary to distinguish this level of reflux.

Reflux - The Disease

Doctors define gastroesophageal reflux *disease* (GERD), as *reflux episodes that cause some sort of measurable problem or consequence*. We are back to careful wording again because now we have to define the words *problem* and *consequence*. Defining *measurable* can also make it tricky.

It is hard for parents to believe that such a common medical problem doesn't have a more precise definition. In June 2001, The North American Society for Pediatric Gastroenterology and Nutrition released official "Guidelines for Evaluation and Treatment of Gastroesophageal Reflux in Infants and Children." This groundbreaking document is the best attempt so far to gather all the knowledge into a single place and give doctors suggested courses of action to follow with their patients. The committee of doctors who wrote the Guidelines defined gastroesophageal reflux disease this way: *Gastroesophageal reflux disease (GERD) occurs when gastric contents reflux into the esophagus or oropharynx [mouth /throat/nose] and produce symptoms.*

The term 'reflux disease' will be used in this book when it is necessary to distinguish this level of reflux.

Squishy Terminology

A very simplistic definition of GERD is easy to understand. But, like the age-old problem of writing a definition for pornography, it can be very tricky to draw the line with words.

Terms you MAY see used to describe **Reflux The Normal Event**	Terms you MAY see used to describe **Reflux The Condition or Illness**	Terms you MAY see used to describe **Reflux The Disease**
▪ Physiologic reflux ▪ Garden variety reflux ▪ Spitting-up ▪ Brits call spitting-up possetting or spilling ▪ Wet burp ▪ Regurgitation ▪ Harmless reflux episodes ▪ Volume reflux of infancy ▪ Non-acid reflux events ▪ Happy spitter ▪ Gastroesophageal Reflux (GER without the word disease added) ▪ Emesis (this is actually a word for the stomach contents)	▪ A touch of reflux ▪ Wait and Watch reflux ▪ Mild reflux ▪ Excessive reflux events ▪ Gastroesophageal Reflux (GER) ▪ Excessive spitting-up ▪ Dr. Sears says, "the Hurting Child"	▪ Gastroesophageal Reflux Disease ▪ GERD (often pronounced to rhyme with bird) ▪ Heartburn (Often used to mean the same as GERD, but it really just describes one particular symptom) ▪ Acid Reflux Disease (this term is often used but is only 99% accurate) ▪ Non-Erosive Reflux Disease (NERD) ▪ Laryngo- Pharyngeal Reflux (LPR)

In real life, reflux does not have neat little boxes with neat little labels that make it clear exactly which box your child fits into.

There is a lot of room for argument over where to draw the line between reflux the event, reflux the condition/illness and reflux the disease. It may be hard to tell which box your baby belongs in.

If your baby has many reflux events and is gaining weight a very slowly, do we call this reflux the condition/illness or reflux the disease? If your baby has many reflux events and is become uninterested in eating, do we call this GER or GERD? And do you call it disease when the number and frequency of episodes is clearly excessive but there is no measurable damage?

Here is a quote from Susan Orenstein, MD in "Pediatric Gastrointestinal Motility Disorders" (1994) about when to call it "reflux disease":

> Since reflux is present in normal individuals, a continuum from normal to diseased exists with respect to gastroesophageal reflux. We should not define reflux disease simply by the deviation from normal values of frequency of duration: we should demand that symptoms, harm, or disability must be produced to meet our definition of disease. This may be difficult to determine, however. Does the patients who has pain induced by acidification, but who does not have histologic esophagitis [damage to the esophagus] or esophageal dysmotility [another type of measurable damage], have reflux disease? If so, it may often be missed. Does the patient who has normal reflux frequency, but who occasionally aspirates refluxate [stomach contents enter the lungs], have reflux disease? Certainly, but this course of events is often extremely difficult to document.

Some people say that you call it disease (GERD) when the baby has *significant* problems and call it a condition when the baby only has *insignificant* problems from the reflux episodes. This is a great idea, but then we are back to defining more squishy words.

In reality, reflux *disease* should probably be called reflux *syndrome*. A syndrome is a medical problem with a whole bunch of different symptoms and each patient has different symptoms.

What Causes Reflux?

The Lower Esophageal Sphincter or the LES for short, is a ring of muscles at the bottom of the esophagus. The LES is supposed to stay contracted or tight, except when your baby swallows or burps. If it opens, the food can backwash up into the esophagus. There are many reasons this can happen.

Here are some common reasons why your baby's food and acid backwash out of her stomach:

Babies tend to eat meals that are very large - a sixteen-pound baby can slurp down a six-ounce bottle with no trouble but a 160-pound man who is ten times larger would probably vomit before managing to consume 60 ounces at a time!

Babies' stomachs aren't as stretchy as adult stomachs and a stiff stomach doesn't contract as efficiently.

Babies tend to flop at the waist, which puts pressure on the stomach and squeezes the food out.

Babies spend a lot of time lying down, often when their stomachs are full so gravity is working against them.

Babies eat a diet of liquids, which bounce up easier than solids.

Babies' digestive systems aren't fully coordinated and the LES at the top of the stomach opens when it doesn't need to.

Babies have a shorter distance from the esophagus to the mouth so a wet burp that only bounces up six inches may end up escaping out of the mouth. This doesn't mean there is more backwash, we just become more aware of it because we have to clean it up.

The amount and frequency of backwash should decrease as your baby guzzles less, her stomach becomes stretchier, her abdominal muscles get stronger, she starts to sit and stand and she starts to eat more solids. As her digestive system and nervous system mature, things will start working smoother, especially the LES.

Researchers have been studying reflux and digestion for a long time. It still isn't completely clear why reflux affects some children but not others. They suspect that acid reflux actually has several possible underlying causes. After all, reflux is really just a fancy term for "vomiting problem" and we all know that vomiting has many causes. It may not really be a single disease/condition - it might be several that look alike.

Parents often tell us theories they have heard about what caused the reflux: long labor, eating spicy food when pregnant, exposure to medications and hysterical mother syndrome. As far as anybody knows, you didn't do anything to make your baby have reflux!

As researchers learn more about the different causes of reflux, they may start to see trends that will help doctors decide which treatment are likely to work best for which child. Currently, treatment focuses on reducing symptoms. Until we understand the disease better, making decisions about the best treatments will take some trial and error.

There is evidence that some families have an inherited form of severe reflux disease. In some families, there is a pattern of multiple generations (siblings, aunts, uncles, grandparents, etc) with severe reflux disease.

If you think your family has a pattern of severe reflux disease, contact the researchers at Allegheny General Hospital, Center for Genomic Science in Pittsburgh and register your family for an ongoing research project. See the resource section at the back of this book for the contact information. You do not need to visit their facility to participate in the project. The interviews and testing are conducted by phone and mail. They can use blood or saliva samples.

After hearing about premature twins with reflux, triplets with reflux and whole families with reflux, we started wondering if it was genetic. At first, all the doctors thought we were crazy, but we convinced a team of geneticists to look at this question. The idea is now widely accepted. Finding the gene could help researchers develop new medications or treatments for children with reflux.

Secondary Causes of Reflux

There are several medical problems that tend to cause reflux. Fixing them can often fix the reflux.

Delayed Stomach Emptying: If your baby's stomach isn't contracting efficiently, food may remain in the stomach without moving into the intestines. Stomachs and intestines have rhythmic contractions just like the heart, and some babies just have poor rhythm.

Prematurity: Premature babies are more likely to have reflux because their digestive systems are not mature and the signals from the brain that control digestion aren't regulated.

Constipation: When the intestines move food too slowly, this can prevent food from leaving the stomach at a normal rate. It is just like the plumbing - if there is a clog somewhere, the whole system backs up.

Hiatal Hernia: A hiatal hernia occurs when part of the stomach protrudes through the diaphragm and into the chest cavity. Food in the top stomach pouch gets squeezed between the lungs with every breath.

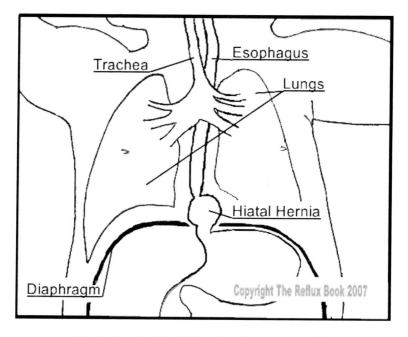

Illustration 4: Hiatal Hernia – the top part of the
stomach is squeezed up into the chest cavity.

Allergies and Intolerances: The stomach rejects the food due to allergies or intolerances.

Neurological or Muscular Issues: Children who have neurological systems or muscles that don't work properly tend to have reflux.

Is Reflux the Same as Colic?

Reflux and colic are very similar. It is easy to mix them up.

Colic is defined as *excessive crying in infancy with no known cause.* Many people believe that colic is a distinct illness, but the term really just means excessive crying. The key is to be sure that there is no treatable cause such as reflux.

When diagnosing colic, doctors use the rule of threes to decide with crying is *excessive*: three hours of crying, three or more days per week, it starts at about three weeks of age and it usually stops fairly suddenly about three months after it started. But this rule doesn't mean that something else like reflux couldn't be causing the excessive crying.

Just a few decades ago, colic was defined as spasms or cramps of hollow internal organs such as the stomach, intestines or kidneys. But researchers who studied crying infants, couldn't find much proof of spasms. Many doctors and parents still believe that some colic is due to intestinal cramps. Many babies with colic behave as if they have severe abdominal pain. They curl up and thrash around. If you hold a baby with colic up against your chest, she will often pull her feet up and kick in a way that makes it look like she is trying to walk up your chest.

One of the most common symptoms of reflux is excessive crying. Researchers believe that many babies with unexplained crying may have reflux, but not all of them. Some may have cramping. Some have excessive gas, which causes cramping. Many doctors believe that colic is due to an immature digestive system that isn't coordinated and doesn't function smoothly. Some babies turn out to be allergic to milk protein. But sometimes, no cause can ever be found. Maybe we aren't looking hard enough or maybe some babies just get upset easily.

> *All of our babies had terrible colic. Now that they are having children of their own, my wife and I joke that all the excessive crying is a sign of high intelligence. My daughter says that her new baby is going to be a genius! Then she mutters about how he had better grow up to save the planet as she paces back and forth with him.*

A researcher studying colic in babies tested the babies for reflux. It was found that 50% of the babies identified as having "colic" also had reflux.

Reflux and colic are different in subtle ways:

Colic	Reflux
Crying more than 3 hours/day, 3 days/week	Crying may occur on and off all day and night.
Happy early in the day with fussiness building as the day goes on.	Often fussy or miserable all day. Some babies are happy with sudden bursts of crying.
Starts at about 3 weeks.	Reflux may be present from birth but may only start to hurt after a few weeks.
Crying is most intense in the evening.	Babies with chronic pain often become overwhelmed at the end of the day and get fussier.
Tends to resolve after 3 months (at about 4 months of age).	Reflux often peaks at 4 months. Crying MAY get significantly better when the baby starts solid foods and sits up but doesn't usually stop overnight.
Parents interpret the crying as digestive pain, but researchers say there is no cause.	Crying is caused by digestive pain. The baby may cry more when fed or after meals or right after burping.
Colic and reflux may exist together. A few parents report their children still have bouts of crying in the evening even though the reflux is under control and all other symptoms are gone.	

When my baby was older, I realized that she probably had colic along with her reflux. The reflux medicines helped a lot, but she still cried every afternoon for a few months.

When your doctor went to medical school, they were probably still teaching the old theory that nervous mothers are the true cause of colic. Yes, mothers of babies with colic do tend to be very nervous and can even be frantic. But the sound of a baby crying for hours on end can be enough to drive the calmest to the edge of sanity.

When the doctor implied that I'm a hysterical new mother and that this is proven to cause colic, I went off on him. I told him in no un-

certain terms that I despite the fact that this is my first baby, I have been around babies all my life and didn't feel the slightest bit nervous till she started crying the previous week and hadn't stopped. I told him that I would be a whole lot more hysterical if he didn't figure out very quickly why my baby was screaming.

Beth's Rule of Sixes

(Completely unscientific)
If you can check any six of these, maybe it isn't "just" colic...

Your baby cries six hours a day
For six days a week
It has been going on for over six weeks
The neighbor six doors down can hear the screaming
You tried six formulas or cut six foods from your diet if nursing
You and your baby need six changes of clothes per day
It takes six hours to feed six ounces
Your baby never sleeps for more than 60 minutes at a time
Your baby spits up six times after each bottle
You keep wondering if you overlooked a 666 birthmark
At the last six appointments doc said "colic" or "babies just cry"
You dread driving anywhere more than six minutes away
Your baby belches like a six year old
Six hours alone with the baby is the maximum anybody can take
You do six loads of laundry a week - just for you and the baby
By six pm, you want a 7&7

Many parents say that intestinal gas is the cause of their baby's colic. Some babies pass a lot of gas with little or no fussing. Other babies seem to be in agony from every bubble. You may be able to help your baby pass the gas quicker by using gravity to advantage. Hot air rises so spending a few minutes with her tush higher than her tummy may help the gas escape. You can also try putting her on her left side for a few minutes and then putting her on her right side. This helps the bubbles move back and forth through the winding intestines. (Remember those toys where you move a marble through a winding maze?)

I come from a family where family meals could be a three-ring circus. My wife's family is the exact opposite – they have "nervous stomachs" and are very certain that proper digestion requires peace. I used to think this was nonsense until we had kids. One kid is very adaptable, but the other kid had terrible colic as a baby and still gets stomachaches after meals if he eats too fast or if there is a lot of commotion. As a baby, he was very upset by having a lot of people around or having his routine disrupted. I used to think it was all in their heads – I think I was wrong. Oddly, now we have a dog that is very good-natured but her stomach won't tolerate any people food (not even one bite) and she starts vomiting if we watch her eat - it makes her nervous. If I want to abuse my stomach by wolfing down large quantities of spicy food, I have to do it at lunch with the guys I work with.

How Common is Reflux?

Harmless reflux episodes are very common in infancy with as many as 50% of otherwise healthy babies spitting up in the first few months of life.

About 20% of babies (one in five) have so many episodes that their parents get a bit worried (reflux the condition). That is a lot of spit up!

A much smaller percentage of children have reflux disease. There are several studies that estimate perhaps 1-8% of children have reflux disease. This comes to several million children in the United States alone. About 2 million children in the US took prescription medicine for digestive problems in 2006.

When we talk with pediatricians at conferences, we often say, "So, do you have many patients with acid reflux?" Some typical responses are: "All of them!" "Doesn't every child have reflux!?!" Or exaggerated eye rolling and a pained facial expression!

Opinions about how many children have reflux have changed dramatically in the past few decades. When doctors first started studying reflux, they thought it only affected adults. By the middle of the last century, reflux was known to exist in children but it was believed to be very rare. The belief was that it only affected a few infants (mostly boys) and mentally handicapped older children. It was believed that all infants stopped refluxing by their first birthday.

We now know that reflux is quite common and can affect children of all ages. In most children, it is a short-term problem lasting a few months.

It is hard to get exact estimates because the definition has changed a lot. Over the years, each study has used a slightly different definition of reflux.

Will My Baby Outgrow Reflux?

It is highly likely your baby will outgrow reflux since approximately 80% of babies outgrow reflux in the first year of life. Many infants show improvement around 4-6 months of age when their digestive systems mature and they are able to sit up independently and control their muscles. Other babies are on the one year or even the two-year plan before their digestive system can manage food gracefully.

At PAGER Association, we have heard every kind of outcome. The babies with "off the charts" severe reflux who are reflux free by the toddler years and the babies with a seemingly mild case who just keep on refluxing into elementary school. We wish there was a way to figure out which babies will have long-term problems and which ones just need time to out-grow reflux. Until then, we encourage all parents to seek medical care and educate themselves regardless of the severity of the symptoms.

> *My Story: When my daughter was diagnosed, the doctor promised it would be gone by six months. At the seven-month check up, the doctor promised it would be gone by nine months. It wasn't and I got more promises. Maybe the doctor was just trying to be nice, but the advice set me up to be disappointed. Another mother told me that there is no firm timetable and this was somehow easier to cope with. I later heard a POW discussing his eight years as a captive. He said that he was always convinced that he would survive but did not set deadlines. He said that the men who convinced themselves that they would be home by the next holiday or birthday set themselves up for an emotional rollercoaster.*

Notes:

2 SYMPTOMS

Your gut tells you something is wrong. Your baby doesn't act like her big sister or the baby next door. You wonder if something could be wrong. The first step to diagnosis and treatment is learning about the symptoms of reflux.

Most children only have a few of the common symptoms you will read about in this chapter. Your child will probably never have any of the serious or scary symptoms. The fact that you are reading this book and learning about the potential problems may actually help your child avoid the worst symptoms and unnecessary discomfort.

Noticing Symptoms

Nobody else spends as much time with your baby and nobody else can see her symptoms as well as you can. It is not surprising that parents are the best observers of their child's symptoms and often notice things about their child that nobody else could possibly notice. Maybe you had a hunch something was not right well before everyone else.

The doctor only spends a few minutes with your baby during check ups so it is important to report what you see at home. All of your little observations are clues for the doctor and may make a huge difference in what your doctor decides to do. The doctor depends on you to provide this information. You are a very important part of your baby's medical team.

> Within a few days of my daughter's birth, I knew something wasn't quite right. Often, I would cry and tell my husband there was something wrong with our baby. Everyone assumed I just had post partum depression. But I listened to my gut and started writing down what I saw that didn't seem right. Instead of telling the doctor, "Something's wrong," I could tell her that my baby woke up crying three times last night and didn't seem hungry and she was very

*fussy during meals this week. Having these facts helped the doctor
realize we were dealing with reflux.*

Most babies have symptoms that start right after birth, but some babies
don't seem to have any trouble right away.

*I had the world's happiest baby. She was so easy to calm and
soothe. At 2 months, she was sleeping 4 and 5 hour stretches. She
never so much as spit up. In comparison to what I had gone through
with my then 2.5-year-old son, she was a dream. I thought that I'd
learned a lot with my first-born and I was reaping the benefits with
my second. Then at 3 months, the reflux started and all hell broke
loose.*

Confusion About Symptoms

Keep in mind that most babies only have one or two symptoms from the
very long list that follows. As you read the following pages, you might
be overwhelmed by the number of other symptoms listed. It may seem
impossible for one disease to have so many different presentations. You
can see why it is sometimes so difficult to recognize reflux.

*The other mom in the waiting room said her son spits up after each
meal but my baby hardly ever needs a burp cloth after a feeding.
How can they both have reflux?*

Some doctors are leaning toward a theory that reflux is not a single disease, but a cluster of symptoms that can have many different causes.
Diseases that have several variations or causes are called heterogeneous.
This term is starting show up in medical journal articles about reflux. It
might explain why there are many confusing and contradictory medical
studies and why no two patients have the same symptoms.

It might be useful to think of reflux as a "syndrome." Syndromes are not
diagnosed based on tests or a short list of mandatory symptoms. They
are diagnosed according to clusters of symptoms and every patient has a
unique set of symptoms.

20

Symptoms Get Worse and Better at Times

It may help to know that your child's symptoms may change a bit from day to day and may change a lot from month to month. Sometimes these changes can be important clues that will help you identify something like a food that bothers her tummy. Other times, the symptoms may just flare up or subside for no reason at all.

An illness such as an ear infection or the stomach flu can cause a temporary disinterest in feeding and an increase in reflux symptoms. Even the eruption of baby teeth with the increase in saliva can cause reflux symptoms to worsen. Sometimes, an illness will cause an older child to stop eating a previously tolerated food. This can be very discouraging if your child is already eating a limited number of foods. It may be necessary to increase the dose of reflux medications for a short period during illnesses. Consult with your doctor.

Parents report that it can take up to one month following an illness for reflux symptoms to abate and eating to return to normal. If your child has been on antibiotics, it is possible that the medication destroyed the good bacteria in the gut and caused stomach distress or diarrhea. Some doctors recommend giving probiotics (beneficial bacteria) to help the body recover quicker.

As reflux starts to go away, the symptoms may stop abruptly or they may go away gradually. Mostly likely, you will see a mix of good days and bad days with the good days gradually outnumbering the bad days. It can be very stressful when a flare-up happens after a quiet week or two and you were starting to think the reflux was gone. The reflux probably *is* going away – just not in nice, neat steps.

Clues and Symptoms of Reflux

These clues are listed vaguely in order from very common to very rare. None of the symptoms are mandatory – not even the common ones. For instance, some babies with significant reflux don't spit up, some don't have any pain and some sleep just fine.

Excessive Spitting up or Vomiting

The common definition of spit-up is a small amount of stomach contents dripping or spiting out of the mouth after a meal. Spitting-up is effortless and the baby may not even notice. The parents are usually much more upset than the baby. Most babies with reflux tend to spit up quite a bit.

> *Our baby just dripped all day long like a leaky faucet. My poor wife kept trying to dress her in those cute outfits – it was a complete waste of time.*

Vomiting is more forceful than spitting-up. Your baby may lose all of her last meal. It may come out of the nose and mouth at the same time. Vomiting may involve gagging, dry heaves and nausea - spitting-up doesn't.

All the spitting and vomiting should start to get better at about six months of age.

There is an easy way to estimate the amount a baby has vomited. Take one ounce of milk or water and pour it on a burp rag or the floor. Note the size of the watermark. One ounce of liquid looks like half a bottle!

In some cases, a baby or toddler may have projectile vomiting. This is a more forceful, often violent form of vomiting. Babies sometimes vomit clear across the room (right onto the new sofa of course). Projectile vomiting is always scary for the parents but it isn't necessarily a serious medical problem.

> *She just vomited. I know she did. I heard it as I walked down the hall with her on my shoulder. I put her down and grabbed a towel from the laundry basket. I looked everywhere. No vomit. Finally, I went into the next room and found the pool of formula I had just fed her. My little 14-pound baby had vomited over 4 feet. We went to the doctor to be sure it wasn't anything dangerous. It was just Olympic worthy reflux.*

Be sure to report vomiting episodes to your doctor just in case it is a sign of a more serious problem such as pyloric stenosis. This is especially important with newborns. Try to report whether your baby loses an entire meal, whether you think she seems "sick," whether she gags and whether the vomiting seemed forceful.

Pain

Reflux can cause pain and may make your baby cry in a variety of ways. She may cry endlessly no matter what you try: holding, feeding or driving in the car. On the other hand, she may be happy most of the time with sudden outbursts of crying or wake up from a deep sleep and cry out. Some babies with reflux are fussy and irritable with short, fleeting periods of happy alertness.

Toddlers may express pain by being extra clingy or fussy with a short frustration tolerance. They are notoriously bad at being able to identify the source of their discomfort and may lash out or switch moods suddenly.

It is painful to be in the same room with a baby who will not stop shrieking, arching her back, clawing and flailing. The piercing pain of a baby who is crying inconsolably can be very distressing to a caretaker. Some babies with severe pain from reflux have been known to cry for hours.

> *She cried so hard and so long that she was hoarse. Her face was red and she was covered in sweat. I was also in tears and completely exhausted. Nothing helped. My husband and I took turns holding her, rocking her, changing her diaper, feeding her and we even gave her a bath. She just would not calm down.*

> *After crying most of the day my neighbor took the baby to her house. I was exhausted and went right to bed. When I opened my window for fresh air, I could hear her screaming from next door.*

Some babies arch their back as a response to pain during eating or reflux episodes. Even though babies may not be very mobile, they can use their strong back muscles to pull away from the breast or bottle. You may notice arching most during mealtime as you both change positions and struggle to find a comfortable position. It may feel like you are baby wrestling rather than providing nourishment. (See Sandifer's Syndrome.)

Remember, not all crying and pain is from reflux. Constipation, milk protein allergy and many other medical conditions can cause pain and crying.

Poor Sleep

Many babies with reflux are such poor sleepers that there is a whole chapter of this book devoted to sleep. Most babies with reflux have some difficulty falling asleep and staying asleep. During sleep, a combination of relaxed muscles (including the stomach muscles) and a reclined sleeping position, allows acid to escape from the stomach and burn the esophagus and mouth.

> *When I took him in for his 4-week checkup, I mentioned to the doctor that he seemed to be crying more and more often especially at night. I asked the doctor if he could have nightmares or night terrors at his age because he would sleep for about an hour and then wake up screaming and did this all night. We soon learned that it was reflux and not night terrors that was causing the night waking.*

Silent or Invisible Reflux

Your baby may not spit up at all. She might just have wet burps, wet hiccups or you might hear food coming part way up her throat. Some parents report that they can hear loud rumbling and strange noises coming from the very tiny digestive systems of their babies. The wet burps and wet hiccups may be quite painful for some babies. Parents learn pretty fast what all of these gurgles and burps mean.

> *When my son refluxes, it sounds like hiccups. If he starts to have a distressed look on his face and his little arms start waving, I know it is time to get ready for the whole meal to come up.*

Silent reflux is the term that doctors use to describe a baby who refluxes but doesn't spit up. The medical term is occult (hidden) reflux. The food and stomach acid come half way up and your baby may swallow hard to keep the stomach contents from getting all the way into her mouth. Your baby may make disgusted faces or cry out suddenly. You may also hear grunting, choking or coughing.

Doctors call this silent reflux. I call it "invisible" reflux since babies who have it are rarely silent. And if you listen closely, you can hear the stomach contents bouncing.

There is some concern that silent/invisible reflux may be under diagnosed and under treated. Without an obvious symptom such as spit-up or vomiting, it may be less obvious that there is a problem. The fact that the stomach contents don't come out of the mouth means there is less laundry, but it can still cause all the same medical problems.

Some babies spit and vomit for months and then stop. In most cases, this means that the reflux is gone, but unfortunately, some of these babies and young children have become silent refluxers.

Poor Eating

Many children with reflux are poor eaters. When they swallow food, it hurts, so they avoid eating. (See the three chapters about feeding for more information.)

Underweight

Reflux can have a big impact on growth. Frequent vomiting or poor feeding can lead to a pattern of slow growth or weight loss.

Your doctor will measure your baby's growth frequently during the course of well baby check-ups. If a worrisome pattern of slow weight gain develops, the doctor may ask you to bring your baby in more frequently for weight checks. Poor weight gain can be a sign that something is wrong. Weight loss of more than a few ounces should be investigated right away.

Gaining the right amount of weight is very important to help your child grow and stay healthy. Very small babies can get in danger quicker if they get sick. (See Failure to Thrive.)

We really had to coax our son to drink a 4-ounce bottle. As soon as he was finished, he would vomit half of it right up. We kept a very close eye on our baby's weight. The pediatrician has us bring him in every other week for weight checks because he had fallen to the fifth percentile. She was concerned that he didn't have enough weight to spare if he got a fever and couldn't eat for a few days. My wife and I really had to work hard to nudge his weight back up past the 5th percentile.

Overweight

Some babies with reflux grow just fine or even become quite over weight. Your baby may have learned that it feels better to have a sip of milk to push the acid back down. From her point of view, she is trying to "fix" the reflux. It is important to watch that she doesn't get her stomach overly full because overeating can aggravate reflux too.

My story: My son was huge! He didn't care a bit when he vomited as long as I fed him again...immediately! The pediatrician urged me to cut him back a bit. It was a fine balance between letting him soothe his sore throat and letting him eat till he threw up – again. Letting him suck a pacifier helped.

Drooling

Immediately after a reflux event, the saliva glands may produce large amounts of saliva to help wash any acid out of the esophagus. You may notice your baby drools a lot even if she is not teething. This is called water brash or hyper-salivation.

I could tell when my baby's reflux was acting up – his shirts would be wet from drooling on them.

Bad Breath

Many babies and children have bad smelling breath when their reflux is acting up. Some parents say that the sour milk smell is one of the easiest clues to monitor.

I'm the father. I'm allowed to have bad breath in the morning. But in our family, it's the baby who could drop a moose at ten paces with her breath. At least it's only bad when her reflux is acting up!

Respiratory Clues and Choking

Not all children with reflux develop breathing problems, but you should be alert to signs of trouble and report any worrisome symptoms to your doctor.

If your baby turns blue or gray, especially around the lips and fingernails, call the doctor immediately. If your can see the spaces between the baby's ribs very clearly when she breathes in, call the doctor.

If your baby is having trouble breathing or stops breathing, call 911 immediately.

Little babies have little airways so any irritation or swelling in the airway can make their breathing sound loud and congested.

A baby with reflux may cough and gag during and after a meal if the meal she just ate is being refluxed back up again and aggravating her airway. She may make throat-clearing noises when this happens.

If acid or acid vapors get all the way into the lungs, it can cause more serious complications such as pneumonia or bronchitis. If your child develops a severe or nagging cough, call your doctor.

If the voice box becomes swollen, your child may get a croupy cough which is a distinctive barking type cough caused by swollen vocal chords. (Most cases of croup are caused by a virus rather than reflux.) Or she can develop stridor, which is a noisy inhale that sounds a bit like Darth Vader.

Babies and children with acid damage to the voice box may have a hoarse or very deep sounding voice. Even babies who don't talk yet can have a hoarse sound to their cry.

Asthma is a constriction of the tubes in the lungs that makes it hard to exhale fully. It may cause a squeaky noise (wheezing), bouts of coughing, shortness of breath or a lack of energy. Asthma symptoms are a bit vague and very easy to miss.

When acid spills into the airway, it can cause swelling and make the tubes in the lungs constrict.

> Jan Gambino wrote an article for Allergy and Asthma Today called, "Noisy Asthma, Silent Reflux." It tells the story of her daughter Rebecca who coughed and wheezed loudly but rarely vomited or showed obvious signs of acid reflux. It took quite a bit of effort to sort out the cause and effect. Once she was aggressively treated for both asthma and reflux, her lungs cleared and she felt much better.

New research shows the most common reason for a patient with reflux to develop asthma may be because the esophagus senses acid headed upward and "warns" the respiratory system to constrict to prevent acid from getting into the lungs. Even acid vapors and droplets in the esophagus are enough to provoke this early warning response in some people.

The connection between reflux and asthma is complicated. Not only can refluxers develop asthma, some asthmatics develop reflux When they are having an asthma attack, their chest muscles heave so much that any food in the stomach starts sloshing around. If your child has symptoms of asthma such as shortness of breath, wheezing, squeaky sounding breathing or bouts of coughing, you should talk to the doctor and read information about asthma. This book will not be enough.

In some people, asthma and reflux symptoms may both be caused by allergies.

Apnea and Apparent Life Threatening Event (ALTE)

Apnea refers to pauses in breathing – usually lasting more than 20 seconds. The traditional definition of apnea is a baby who sleeps so deeply, her brain forgets to keep her breathing at an even rate.

Call 911 IMMEDIATELY if your baby stops breathing for more than 20 seconds.

An Apparent Life Threatening Event or ALTE is a prolonged apnea event. Many doctors define an ALTE as any event that scares the parents.

There is some evidence that reflux causes some apnea episodes and some ALTEs, but more research is needed.

Even if your baby starts breathing again and seems fine it is vital to have a complete medical evaluation and determine the cause of the breathing problems. It is important to call 911 immediately.

> *It was the longest moment of my life. She started choking and then she just went limp. I turned her over and patted her back. She started breathing but she was pale and weak. Something was terribly wrong. I was so scared I could hardly dial the phone to call 911.*

One possible cause of an ALTE can be closed vocal cords (larynx). During a reflux event, the body tries to protect the airway by shutting the vocal cords, which closes off the airway. When the chords close for a few seconds, this is. It prevents acid from spilling into the airway. Occasionally, the vocal cords stay shut after the reflux is cleared. This is bad. It is called a laryngospasm and is the main cause of "awake apnea" spells. The baby may look surprised and then become limp and pale with blue lips.

Even brief pauses in breathing can be a problem if the baby also has a pale or grey look to their face, blue lips or blue fingernails. All worrisome signs like this need to be reported to the doctor immediately.

> *At 5 months of age, my daughter had a cough and a stuffy nose. I noticed that her lips were turning blue when I nursed her but her color returned to normal when she stopped nursing. I called the doctor right away and I was told to bring her in. Of course, when I got there, her color was normal but the doctor explained that he was glad I came in and wanted to watch her closely for a few hours.*

Parents worry terribly after their baby has experienced an apnea event or ALTE. Even though the baby has received a full evaluation and a clean bill of health, parents often feel a need to monitor their babies in case it happens again. Parents often beg the doctor for an apnea monitor (a device to signal when a baby pauses or stops breathing). If they don't have a machine to help monitor their baby, these parents become "human apnea monitors," sleeping with one eye open or the baby monitor strapped to their pillow at the highest volume. This can be a dangerous situation when the parents get so tired they can't function. We know parents who have driven off the road because they never sleep.

Ear, Sinus and Throat Infections

Doctors who treat sinus and ear infections recently had the inspiration to look at reflux as a possible cause of these infections when no other reason could be found.

If acid gets into the sinuses, it can remove the mucus that helps defend her from viruses and leave her vulnerable to colds and sinus infections. When an adult refluxes, the back of the mouth (soft palate) rises to block acid from squeezing up into the nose and sinuses. In babies, the soft palate may not do the job properly and your baby may vomit out of her nose. This is extremely painful.

Some babies get acid up into their nose so far that it can flow into the Eustachian tubes that run from the nose to the ears, pooling behind the eardrum. There is some evidence that acid may cause burning ear pain.

Some ear, nose and throat doctors believe that reflux can cause ear infections. (Illustration 1 shows the Eustachian tubes.)

> *My son with reflux kept getting ear infections. The doctor said to keep him as upright as possible when feeding him and after meals so the milk wouldn't flow from the back of his throat into his ear tubes. It helped a bit.*

Some children may have enlarged or infected tonsils due to reflux. At least one doctor has found that removing chronically infected tonsils seems to help calm the reflux – perhaps by eliminating the pus, which drains down the throat and causes nausea?

Sandifer's Syndrome

Sandifer's Syndrome is a term for neck or back spasms caused by acid reflux. Other terms for this condition include torticollis (head tilting to one side) and dystonia (muscle spasms that last a long time). Sometimes, the movements associated with Sandifer's Syndrome look like seizures so a doctor may refer a baby to a neurologist or the Emergency Room for evaluation. If testing rules out actual seizures, treatment for reflux may be recommended.

In recent years, some doctors have used the term Sandifer's Syndrome to describe deliberate arching and thrashing movements that babies make when they are in pain, but the original definition of Sandifer's Syndrome only included muscle spasms of the back and neck, not deliberate movements.

Esophageal Damage

Even though we hear a lot about esophageal damage in the media, it is not common in children. It is more likely for children to experience pain with no damage. Doctors call this visceral hyper-algesia. (Translates to gut+super+pain.)

> *I was sure she had esophagitis or an ulcer like my grandfather. Her long bouts of crying had to be from more than just reflux but the tests didn't show any damage to her esophagus. The doctor explained that her esophagus lining is hyper sensitive.*

Your baby's esophagus is very sensitive to acid and may become red and swollen (esophagitis) when exposed to acid. Very rarely, the lining may develop raw spots called ulcers. If the ulcers bleed, the child may vomit blood or pass dark, tarry stools that look like coffee grounds and smell terrible. In rare cases, children can become anemic from losing too much blood.

Strictures, a webbed type of scar tissue, may form when esophageal damage heals. The strictures may partially block the esophagus causing food to get stuck on the way down to the stomach.

Tooth Enamel Erosion

Tooth enamel may be damaged from acid reflux. If your child sleeps very deeply at night, she might not wake up during a reflux event and the acid can pool in the mouth and damage the teeth. This can be mild damage to the surface of the teeth or serious tooth damage. Other signs that your baby's teeth are at risk for damage include bad breath and constant drooling. See a dentist early and keep a close eye on your baby's teeth

Behavioral Issues

Poor sleep and chronic discomfort can cause your little one to be whiny or clingy. Some toddlers may become hyperactive, angry or aggressive. A few become overly passive.

> I could always tell when her medication needed to be increased. She is normally very sweet and affectionate so it was obvious something was wrong when she would cry for no reason and push me away. Once the medication was increased, she went back to her normal, happy personality.

Dysphagia or Swallowing Problem

Almost all babies gag and splutter occasionally during a meal. A baby with reflux may do this at every meal. It may seem that she can't settle into a good feeding pattern and you both have to start and stop frequently.

People think that all babies know how to eat from the moment they are born. Most babies do, but not premature babies and not some babies with reflux. Eating actually involves 20-30 small steps and is much more complicated that most people realize. Some babies need more time to figure it out or may need help from a swallowing specialist.

Dysphagia is a fancy word for a swallowing problem. Dysphagia is difficulty coordinating sucking, breathing and swallowing. A baby may develop an abnormal pattern of sucking and swallowing because of reflux pain or the dysphagia have an underlying cause such as prematurity or respiratory disease.

A baby with dysphagia may experience coughing and gagging during meals. Over time, a baby or toddler with dysphasia may become fearful of trying new textures and foods.

Some people with reflux experience esophageal spasms or cramps which make them feel that food is stuck half way down their esophagus. These spasms can be quite painful.

Sensory Issues

Some infants and toddlers develop a sensitivity to the touch, taste and smell of food because of long-term feeding problems from reflux disease. Feeding involves processing all of the sensory information and making sense of it. If pain has been associated with feeding, it is possible for the sensory system to under-react or over-react to food.

A child may appear upset or agitated if someone touches in or around the mouth or even the cheeks and chin. Attempts to touch the mouth or put textured food in her mouth will often result in crying, avoidance, choking and vomiting. A speech therapist or an occupational therapist who specializes in infant feeding problems may be consulted to evaluate the nature of the sensory problem and offer treatment to normalize the sensory processing system. Most speech therapists and occupational therapists do not work with feeding issues so you may have to consult local gastroenterologists to find one who does. It is important to get help early if you suspect a problem.

Delayed Milestones

An infant who has experienced pain with eating may be slow to develop feeding skills. Another baby with reflux may be so fussy, there is no time to practice motor skills or develop play skills. The good news is that when the pain from reflux goes away, most infants and toddlers quickly catch up. If your baby seems to be lagging behind, talk to the pediatrician and ask for a developmental check-up.

Free developmental checks are available in each state through the local school system or health department. Early Intervention serves children birth to 3 years and Child Find serves children 3-5 years. Any parent or physician may call and ask for a full developmental screening if there are concerns about any area of development (speech, movement, feeding, hearing, etc). All services are free to all residents of the United States.

Symptoms? Signs? Sequelae?

If you read medical journals, it may help to know that there are several medical terms that basically mean "diagnostic clue." A "symptom" is the term used for things the patient must tell the doctor because they aren't visible (like headaches). A "sign" is the medical term for things that doctors can observe but the patient might not notice (like an odd color to the skin.). A "sequela" is a consequence. (This Latin word is pronounced suh-QUELL-uh. The plural is pronounced the same but spelled sequelae.)

The terms are confusing and everybody mixes them up. When a doctor sees a child spit up several times during the visit, the spitting up can be considered a "sign." If the doctor doesn't see the spit up but mom reports it, do we then call it a "symptom?" And what about poor weight gain? It is probably most correctly a consequence or sequela of reflux, but it appears on every list of "symptoms" of reflux because it is an important diagnostic clue.

Notes:

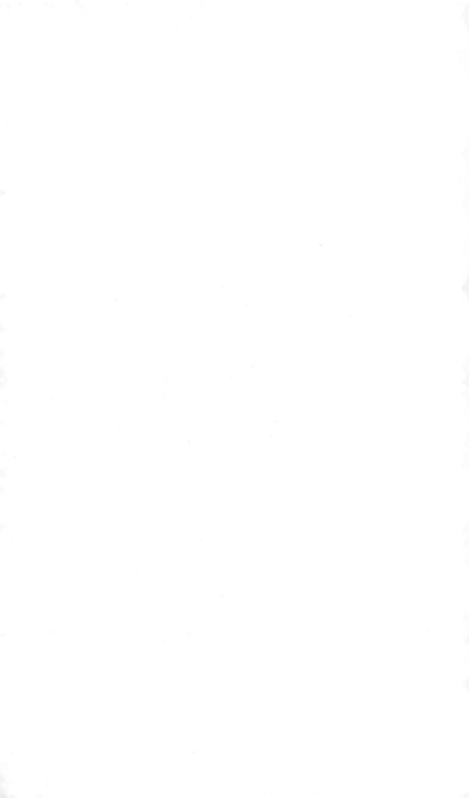

3 DIAGNOSIS

Reflux is usually diagnosed after the doctor listens to the parents and examines the baby. The North American Society of Pediatric Gastroenterology, Hepatology and Nutrition (NASPGHAN) feels that few children need to be tested. Not doing any tests may seem odd to you, but it is standard procedure.

If the doctor determines that a test is needed, you are encouraged to go to the Testing Chapter for detailed information on everything from how to prepare your little one to what will happen during the test.

In the past, reflux was believed to be extremely rare, leading to under-diagnosis of the condition. Now we realize that reflux is very common and there is some debate about whether it is being over-diagnosed or over-treated. Not every child who has reflux events needs a diagnosis and most don't need to be treated with medication.

When you are talking to the doctor about reflux, keep in mind that there are many reasons for a baby to cry, spit up or vomit. Reflux is just one of them. Along with reflux, doctors and parents need to consider constipation, allergies and many other possible causes.

Suspecting the Diagnosis

Getting a diagnosis of reflux depends on two factors – somebody needs to first notice symptoms and then they need to be familiar with the concept of reflux in children and realize it might be the explanation.

If your baby spits up excessively and cries a lot, the idea of reflux might have come up early – maybe even in the hospital.

The nurse at the hospital said my two-day-old baby seemed to be spitting-up quite a bit and getting fussy after eating. She said to expect a few rough months. I wish she had told me more. It would have been nice to know the word "reflux" – I would have looked it up.

Perhaps your pediatrician was the first to suggest reflux when you reported common symptoms such as excessive spitting up or excessive crying.

I called the pediatrician because I was worried about how much my baby was spitting up and how she would cry for an hour afterward. He told me that he could probably diagnose acid reflux on the phone that night, but he had me bring her in the next day just to make sure it wasn't a virus.

Sometimes even strangers can diagnose a baby with reflux. Occasionally, reflux can be diagnosed at a distance.

I was somewhat famous at the grocery store since my first daughter spit up constantly. When I came in with my new baby, the guy who mops the floors only needed one look at the jumbo burp rag and the spit-up all over my shirt. He knew the drill. He grabbed his mop and got ready to clean the floors behind us. I knew it was time to call the doctor.

You may have noticed that your baby had symptoms of reflux, but you may not have known that they were signs of a problem. Unless you were familiar with the concept that babies can have reflux, you would have no reason be suspicious.

I had never spent much time around other babies. Somehow, I didn't realize that her 24/7 crying and spitting-up wasn't normal.

Other symptoms patterns may take longer to notice or appear. Some babies don't begin to experience pain or discomfort for many weeks.

Things were fine during the first few weeks. He spit up but never cried. Then the acid started to hurt and by the second month, he was screaming nonstop.

If your baby or child has less common symptoms such as pneumonia or sinus infections, it may take many months before anybody starts to think about the role of reflux. The most unusual symptoms such as tooth enamel damage may be so subtle that they are missed for years.

My son had such unusual symptoms of reflux that we didn't even start talking about a diagnosis until he was more than a year old and had three bouts with pneumonia. We always assumed his respiratory illnesses were due to colds and viruses.

Some parents have a very strong instinct that something is 'wrong' but they may not completely trust their own instincts.

Everybody told me that I was being overly worried. They kept saying that all babies spit up and all babies cry. But it never seemed right to me that my son never had a peaceful moment. I just knew it wasn't right but I didn't listen to my heart and my baby suffered for a long time. I should have brought up my suspicions a month ago.

Going to the Doctor

Your pediatrician or family doctor is probably going to be the one to diagnose and treat your child's reflux. Most babies and toddlers have reflux that is easy to diagnose and responds to the standard treatments, so they don't need to see a pediatric gastroenterologist.

The first person to talk to about your suspicion of reflux is your child's doctor. You may want to schedule an appointment to discuss your concerns and list the symptoms you see. Often, your child's doctor will feel comfortable making a diagnosis of reflux just by asking you a lot of questions.

Sometimes parents tell us that the doctor doesn't seem concerned about a parent's report of symptoms during a well check-up. Your concerns about reflux can get lost when there are so many other topics to cover during a well check-up such as shots and car seat safety. I often tell parents to schedule a separate "sick visit" just to address the concerns of feeding and digestion.

Guidelines for Diagnosis

Guidelines for the Evaluation and Treatment of Gastroesophageal Reflux in Infants and Children were written by the North American Society of Pediatric Gastroenterology, Hepatology and Nutrition (NASP-

GHAN). Parents and professionals can get copies by calling NASPGHN at the number in the resource list. This professional association of pediatric gastroenterologists does not recommend testing for babies with typical reflux unless they have unusual symptoms, "warning signs" of other diseases, significant complications of acid reflux, or they don't respond to treatment.

> *"In most infants with vomiting, and in older children with regurgitation and heartburn, a history and physical examination are sufficient to reliably diagnose GERD, recognize complications and initiate management." Journal of Pediatric Gastroenterology and Nutrition. 2001;Vol 32: Supplement 2, 1-31.*

Trial of Treatment to Diagnose Reflux

Some babies may have symptom patterns that are not quite clear. Even after talking with you about reflux, the doctor may not be quite sure if your baby has it. One simple way of confirming that your baby has reflux is to start treating her as if she has reflux and see if it helps.

Trying a treatment to confirm a diagnosis is called *empiric* treatment. The Latin and Greek roots of the word empiric are related to the terms try, experience, knowledge and skill.

Some parents may feel that this is an unscientific way of making a diagnosis, but it is actually quite common in the field of medicine. Pediatricians often find they must guess what is wrong with children who are too young to tell them. When it comes to reflux, empiric treatment is a practical and acceptable approach.

You may be told to try several home care treatments for a week or so and report on whether they help. You can read all about Home Care and Positioning in the chapter on that topic. The doctor may also give your baby medication to see if that makes a difference. There are two chapters on Medication that you can read.

Myths

Some old ideas about reflux can interfere with getting a proper diagnosis. All of these ideas were believed to be true in the past. Now we know they are all false.

Only babies have reflux
All babies with reflux outgrow it by their first birthday
All babies with reflux spit-up a lot
Happy spitters can't have serious reflux
The only important symptoms are spitting-up, poor weight gain and pneumonia.
Babies don't experience real pain like adults
If a child is hungry, she will eat
Reflux always responds to medicine

Notes:

4 TREATMENT OVERVIEW

There are many different types of treatments that can be helpful for reflux. There are full chapters on various treatments.

Home Care and Positioning – Chapter 5
Feeding Tips for Babies – Chapter 6
What to Feed Your Baby – Chapter 7
Medications – Chapter 8
Giving Medications – Chapter 9
Reflux in Older Children – part of Chapter 15
Feeding Your Older Child – Chapter 16
Feeding Clinics, Tube Feeding and Surgery – in Chapter 17
Alternative Medicine – Chapter 18

This chapter is not about the treatments. This chapter helps you understand how doctors decide whether your baby will need any treatment and how they decide what treatments to try next.

Expect Improvement, not Perfection

The goal of treatment for reflux is to control pain and other symptoms. In the next few chapters, you will read a great deal about strategies for *reducing* acid, vomiting or pain through various treatments such as positioning, medication and diet.

The treatments rarely *cure* reflux. The reflux usually goes away by itself in time. Meanwhile, gaining control over symptoms is often enough to allow your baby to thrive and allow you to concentrate on everyday parenting tasks. In time, most babies respond to a combination of treatments and begin to feel better. Most treatments for reflux do not have dramatic results. It is more common for the symptoms to get better gradually over a period of days or weeks.

This book provides a complete guide to possible treatments because there is no "one size fits all" treatment for reflux. In some parts of the country, one treatment is more popular and in a different part of the country, another treatment is more popular. This can add to the confusion for parents as they gather information about treatments for reflux from doctors, friends and the internet.

Wait and See

Babies who have *reflux the condition* may not need treatment. If your baby is growing and looks and acts well, the doctor might recommend observing your baby and seeing if she manages the symptoms without intervention. Many children with reflux don't need any treatment. It is likely your doctor will ask you to bring the baby in more frequently to monitor the reflux. Your doctor is also counting on you to report any changes.

If your doctor wants to wait before starting treatment and you disagree, be sure to discuss the situation with the doctor. Perhaps you could keep a journal and write down symptoms and patterns that you are seeing at home. Some babies act and look fine at the doctor's office and then scream and cry all night.

If your baby has moderate symptoms, you may find yourself wanting to put off medical treatment at first but then change your mind later. Or, you may feel that you can just tough it out and wait for your baby to out grow reflux using home care techniques without medicine. If your baby is in pain, it might not be fair to make her wait. You and your doctor might have this conversation several times before making a treatment decision.

Treat Other Causes of Crying

Babies cry to communicate their needs. We often wish they could be more specific in their communication! Since babies cannot tell us exactly what is wrong, parents and doctors are left guessing what the source of the discomfort is. A baby may have one or many pain issues such as ear infections, colic or constipation along with reflux.

Some babies are *high need* and seem to be more easily distressed by noise and other environmental factors. Be sure you and the doctor have addressed other reasons for crying and distress before focusing just on reflux as the cause for all pain. There are many books on calming and comforting a fussy baby. Some parents have had a great deal of success with techniques from these books.

One Step at a Time

It is best to try one new treatment at a time and evaluate the success of each change. A doctor may gradually introduce new treatments such as diet, positioning and step-up the strength of the medication gradually in an attempt to find a treatment plan that controls symptoms.

It often takes a bit of trial and error to find the best treatment plan. It may seem as if the doctor is randomly writing another prescription or handing over a formula sample. In reality, the doctor is going through a systematic process of evaluating the symptoms and adding one treatment at a time until the symptoms are under control.

At times it might be necessary to start with strong medication or tests and gradually step-down the treatment once they have controlled the symptoms. Unfortunately, the doctors do not have a test to guide them in predicting which child needs the full strength, aggressive treatment and which child needs the home care/wait and see option. You and the doctor may not always agree on what to do next.

If you follow the treatment plan, watch your baby carefully and report to the doctor, this helps the doctor make good decisions about adjusting the treatment.

Adjusting the Treatment Plan

As your baby begins to feel better, you may wonder if the treatment is still necessary. If you are using an expensive formula or medication, you may wish there was an alternate that was less costly. If your baby is on a strong medication or on a medication with side effects, you may be motivated to decrease or eliminate the medication if it isn't needed. If you are using positioning therapy that is a hassle, you may be waiting for the day you can stop using it. While it is tempting to make adjustments at home, it is vital to consult the doctor before modifying the treatment plan.

At some point, the doctor may ask you to stop treatment for a few weeks or a month and observe if symptoms return. This is a way for the doctor to figure out whether treatment is still needed. It can be particularly helpful when your baby has very confusing symptoms and reactions to medications. Stopping the treatment can be as a type of test to figure out what is happening.

> *We had tried all the medicines and increased the dose several times. I was completely appalled when the doctor said we needed to get him off all meds for a week and see what was really going on – we had made too many changes to know. I was scared to death to do this and shocked when it worked. The crying stopped. The best we can figure, he must have been having side effects from the medication - like a headache.*

Some children have reflux symptoms that disappear and then reappear for short periods. A few parents report that the reflux reappears after an illness or during a growth spurt. A few of these children need medication for a few weeks or even a few months during growth spurts. If a baby or child exhibits new symptoms, you will need to consult the doctor again for advice and recommendations. The treatments may change as your baby gets older.

Remember: Do not try any positioning, diet, medication or other treatment without first consulting with your doctor. You might feel knowledgeable about reflux and be tempted to stop, start or change a treatment on your own. It is always best to consult with the doctor either by phone or during an office visit before changing the plan. Even over-the-counter medicines need to be approved by the doctor.

Notes:

5 HOME CARE AND POSITIONING

At home, you may need to care for your baby in special ways to sooth the pain from reflux and help her feel better. All of the caretaking is centered on keeping your baby comfortable, keeping her upright and avoiding things that trigger symptoms.

Most babies with "normal reflux" and "reflux the condition" will respond to these home care techniques and not need any other treatment. Babies with "reflux the disease" will probably need medication as well as positioning and home care. Don't stop the home care if you start medication. Doing both can be very beneficial.

Through trial and error, you have probably figured out some ways to feed and care for your baby throughout the day. There is an important reason why you do each thing - your baby has communicated to you what she likes and needs. This is home care. This chapter will give you many ideas to try. Only your baby can tell you which ones help her.

We each found our own little ways to help her. Daddy got really good at waltzing to soothe her and I specialized in the swaddling. As she grows, we watch for new ideas and adjust what we do.

Avoid Exposure to Smoke

Exposure to smoke has been proven to aggravate reflux, so do not allow anybody to smoke around your child or wear clothes that smell like smoke. Ask your doctor for a prescription that says, "No smoking around the baby," and post it where all can see.

```
                              303
Name. . . . . . . . . . . . . . . . . . . . . . . . . . . . . . . . . . . .  Age . . . . .

Address. . . . . . . . . . . . . . . . . . . . . . . . . . . .  Date. . . . . . . .

℞   Do NOT smoke around                                          506

      this child
510
  Units _____

  Refills  NR  1  2  3  4  5

  Void after: _____
                                                                    304
  ☐ Do Not Substitute      _____
                                        Signature
```

Soothing

Many babies with reflux spend a great deal of their day fussing and crying from pain. If your baby is in a lot of pain, finding ways to soothe her may consume your day.

> *I feel like I spend every minute comforting her. I hardly have time to get a glass of water or answer the phone. I wish she could sit in ANY of her brand new baby equipment. It is just sitting here gathering dust while I hold her.*

Swaddling: Swaddling is an age-old technique to make a baby feel safe and secure. Use a light, stretchy blanket to wrap your baby firmly. The arms are generally wrapped to prevent them from jerking and startling the baby. There are many videos on the internet or ask your doctor.

Movement: Swaying, gently rocking in a rocking chair, or a car ride may sooth a crying baby. A device that vibrates the crib on infant seat may be a lifesaver. Walking back and forth across the room is most common way to keep your baby moving. Dr. Karp recommends a special type of jiggling in his videos and books.

Distraction: Some babies respond well to being distracted – it helps them think about something other than their pain. When your baby gets fussy, take her to another room and try another position or positioning device. Take her out to the park. Put on some fun music.

One day I found that I could calm her by standing in front of the mirror. We were quite a sight! Her face was red from crying and she was wearing a dirty outfit. I was a mess with barely brushed hair and bloodshot eyes. But we broke the cycle of crying and had a few minutes of fun.

◆

My husband likes to play "airplane" with our son. Our son squeals with delight while perched on my husband's outstretched arms. It drives me crazy to watch him since I am so careful to move slowly and gently. Sometimes the "airplane" spits-up but everyone enjoys this activity so much that it is worth it.

A warm bath may be distracting and it might relax her. Get in with her and use this as playtime or relaxation.

Fresh air and bright light may make her sleepy. Or, she might be interested in having a look around.

Loose Clothing: Make sure the diaper is loose and her waistbands aren't too tight or uncomfortable. Some parents routinely loosen the diaper after a feeding so it doesn't squeeze the stomach, which can trigger reflux episodes.

Sucking: Many babies with reflux feel better when they are allowed to suck constantly. Sucking helps push any stomach acid back down into the stomach. It also signals the body to produce more saliva, which can help wash the acid down.

Sucking on the breast or a bottle may help, but can also encourage your baby to overfill her tummy and cause more reflux episodes. Sucking on something that doesn't fill her tummy may be helpful. Most parents use pacifiers but you can also let her suck your thumb, offer a bottle with a very small hole in the nipple or offer a breast that is mostly empty. Some babies will accept a small sip of water to wash down the acid.

My little gerdling was addicted to her pacifiers. My other baby never learned to use one but she would insist on having at least three in her sight at all times. We put several in her crib every night.

White Noise: many babies with reflux respond well to the noise of a fan, the washing machine or running water. The easiest way to get white noise is to buy radio or alarm clock that has environmental noises like rain or buy a CD with soothing noises. The sound of a heartbeat is particularly soothing to some babies.

Positioning

Positioning is an important form of treatment for reflux. It means keeping your baby's body positioned so that gravity is working with you to help keep her stomach contents from seeping out. Think of your baby as a funny jug with a leaky top and a rounded bottom. You want to keep it upright most of the time but it won't stand up by itself so you need to figure out other ways to keep it from tipping over.

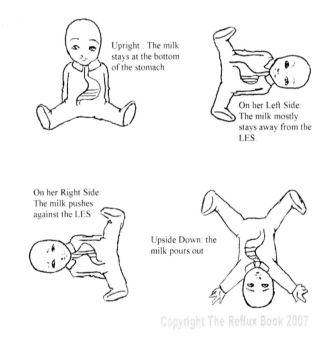

Illustration 5: *These pictures show the liquid in your baby's stomach when she is upright (best), when she is laying on her left side (good), when she is laying on her right side (not good), and upside down (worst).*

48

There is an abundance of baby gear on the market today. Rather than go out and buy an expensive item, it might be possible to get advice from another parent or borrow an item before purchasing it. Sharing information and experiences on baby equipment is a favorite topic on the PAGER Association discussion board

Observe your baby closely for clues about which gear might work best. If you baby likes motion, look at the hammock or crib vibrators. If your baby really likes being upright, look at devices that will help her sleep safely in an upright position.

The American Academy of Pediatrics recommends that parents not use any type of positioning device because they don't feel devices are helpful, necessary or safety tested.

Most parents of children with reflux rely heavily on positioning devices and feel that they are very helpful. Be very careful with the devices you choose and talk to your doctor about safety.

Holding

Keeping a baby upright for 30 minutes after a meal may reduce reflux symptoms. Some babies seem to be more comfortable when held upright most of the day.

This is hard work. You and your back need a break. Be sure to let dad, grandma or a neighbor take a turn holding the baby. And somebody may discover a new position that helps your baby feel better.

Minimize bouncing and jostling: Train yourself not to bounce her up and down, especially after a meal when her stomach is full. Sway instead.

Reduce the pressure on her stomach: Some babies with reflux hate to have pressure on their tummies. She might prefer to be against your chest rather than over your shoulder. If she is slumped over your shoulder it can put too much pressure on her tummy.

Try the Colic Hold : Some babies with reflux or gas like pressure on their stomachs. Lay her down with her tummy on your arm and her legs hanging down on each side of your arm. You can hold her with her head in the crook of your elbow or with her head in your hand. Figure out which feels safer for you and keep her head elevated a bit. Swaying while holding can help.

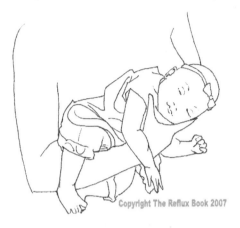

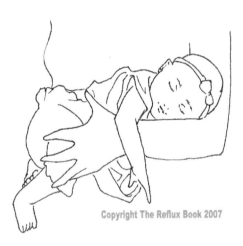

Illustration 6: *The Colic Hold*

Wearing Your Baby

You may find that using a fabric baby carrier is the best option to save your back and keep your baby comfortable. It may take a few tries to find the best style. This is a great way to keep her upright after a meal.

If you use a front carrier, you may have to adjust the carrier to keep your baby from slouching too much. She may feel more comfortable if the carrier comes all the way up to her armpits so the top edge is higher than her stomach and isn't putting pressure on the stomach. Putting your baby in the carrier face out lets her see the world but it can put pressure on her tummy. When your baby is very young, she may be too floppy to sit well in the front carrier. Try again in a few weeks.

Some babies with reflux love the semi reclining position of a sling. Other babies hate it because they are leaning back and they are in a slumping position. Try positioning her a bit more upright and see if this helps or try a different brand of sling. You may find that she is more comfortable in the sling when she is turned a bit onto her left side.

Upright Seating

Once your baby has good head and trunk control and can almost sit up by herself, she might like an entertainment center/saucer or a high chair. It is important for her to have good control so she doesn't slide down or slump over and put pressure on her stomach. A high chair can be a nice play surface for a baby who is very active and needs to stay in place a few minutes to digest a meal before resuming her busy schedule of crawling, climbing and spitting.

There are a variety of pillows intended to help support your baby when she is almost ready to sit up by herself.

Baby Seats, Bouncers and Swings

There are a variety of baby seats and bouncers available in every baby store. A seat that keeps her legs straight and prevents pressure on her stomach will provide the most comfort to her stomach.

Many babies are more comfortable with the most upright seats. Most bouncer seats lean back too far and are not as comfortable because the reclining position can actually provoke reflux. You can try tilting a seat by placing folded towels under it.

If your baby likes the infant seat, it may be tempting to keep her in it as she gets older. Eventually she will be able to squirm and tip it over. You don't want the seat to be on a table the day she learns this trick.

Your baby might enjoy sitting in a swing. Turning on the swing may not be a good idea – the motion may increase the reflux. Some swings let you adjust the seat to a more upright position.

Studies show that some babies have more reflux episodes when they are in an infant seat or bouncer. You need to watch your baby closely to see if the sitting position helps or makes things worse.

Did you know that infant seats were originally designed for spitty babies? They were called Chalasia (kuh - LAY- zhuh) Chairs. Chalasia is an old word for loose sphincter or reflux.

Tummy Time

When an infant has to spend additional time upright due to reflux, it may seem like there is no time to place her on her stomach. With the "back to sleep" campaign many babies are spending more time than ever on their backs during the first months of life. Some babies even develop a bald/flat spot on the back of their head.

Try to place your baby on her stomach a few times every day, even if it is just a moment or two. When your baby is on her tummy, she is using her arm and shoulder muscles and they will get stronger. It also helps her hands become strong and learn to grip.

If she is prone to spitting - up when she is on her stomach, try to have tummy time before a meal. She may enjoy looking at you if you lie down beside her or place her on a wedge. Looking at her cute little face in the mirror may be an enjoyable activity. Another idea is to ask dad to be in charge of playtime or tummy time. It may be very beneficial to everyone.

At first, she may cry and protest because this position may seem so new to her. If she really hates it, don't torture her. Try again another time.

Diaper Changes

If your baby cries or protests with every diaper change, it may indicate that she is refluxing when she is placed on her back. You may find you need to elevate the changing table so she is never flat during diaper or clothing changes. You may need a changing table wedge. It is extremely important to use a safety strap and to stay beside your baby every moment she is on the changing table.

You can also try diapering your baby while she is lying on her tummy by rolling her from side to side. It takes practice. A few parents have even figured out how to keep their baby completely upright during diaper changes – this usually involves two adults but may be worth the effort.

Car Seats

Car seats are designed to hold a baby securely during car rides. Some parents of babies with reflux find that a car seat can do much more than that. In the olden days, before all of the baby gear was invented, parents of refluxers were told to let their babies sleep and play in a car seat to maintain an upright position.

If a car seat is meeting your needs and not causing an increase in reflux symptoms, there is no need to make any changes. Just remember to let her out to try other positions and get some exercise. There is some concern about keeping a child in a sitting position too much of the day – her head might end up flat on the back and she won't get to practice using her abdominal and back muscles.

If your baby cries while she is in the car seat, it is possible that the reclining position of the car seat is causing her to reflux. You might want to try a more upright model or you might just have to delay the long trip to grandma's house until she is feeling better. Traveling at night is one way to avoid a very long and loud car ride.

The typical infant car seat may place a great deal of pressure on the stomach. It might help to place a small receiving blanket in the base of the seat so her hips are elevated slightly and there is less of a bend in the seat. This takes some pressure off the stomach.

If your baby chokes or vomits a lot in the car seat, it might distract you so much that you drive dangerously. If possible, have another adult sit in the back with your baby.

One day she choked in rush hour traffic. I hit the flashers, crossed three lanes and pulled over in one smooth move. Then I found I couldn't get her seat straps undone. I panicked before I realized it was easier to unbuckle the whole seat and tip it over. Disaster averted. My husband couldn't believe how calm I was about it. Look out NASCAR, here I come! We bought a different car seat that was more upright and she hasn't choked since then.

Sleep Positioning

The goal of sleep positioning is to elevate the sleep surface so the head is higher than the rest of the body This section describes what you need to know about different ways to keep your little one on an elevated surface.

A Word About Safety

Before you elevate the crib or bassinet, be sure you have asked the doctor if elevating the sleep surface is recommended for your baby.

When you read the descriptions of products available such as wedges and hammocks, you might think that it would be easier to just make something yourself. But it is hard to make something that is really safe. With any modification to the sleep surface, inspect every inch for safety: strangulation hazards, suffocation, pinch points or the entire thing falling apart or tipping over.

American Academy Of Pediatrics Sleep Position Statement

The American Academy of Pediatrics has issued a recommendation that all babies be placed on their backs to sleep. New studies indicate the risk of SIDS is greater for the average baby than the risk of choking. But there are clearly a very small number of babies who do tend to choke from reflux when laying flat on their backs. In fact, one of the oldest treatments for reflux was to have the baby sleep face down with her head elevated.

The AAP Guidelines used to state that babies with reflux were exempt from this recommendation. In 2005, the AAP dropped the exemption for babies with reflux and now insists that all babies sleep on their backs. If you have seen your child choking while on her back, please have a long talk with your baby's doctor.

The American Academy of Pediatrics has not tested or approved any of the sleeping devices described below. They recommend that babies be placed on their backs, in a separate bed with a firm surface, in their parents' room, with a pacifier. Babies should be dressed lightly so they don't overheat.

We recognize that many parents of children with reflux report extreme difficulty getting enough sleep. Quite a few parents feel it is safer to do what ever is necessary to get some sleep than to be exhausted and lose their temper or drive the whole family into a ditch the next day. We know plenty of parents sleep in recliners or sitting up on a pile of pillows with their baby on their chest. Unfortunately, that may be the only way to get an hour or two of precious sleep. If this describes your family, talk to your doctor about safe sleeping.

Raising the crib

Raising the head of the crib may help your baby reflux less and sleep better. For some babies, raising the bed is highly effective but other babies don't respond to this treatment. Raising the bed a few inches may help. Raising it to a 30 or 45-degree angle may produce better results.

If you use a steep angle, you will find your baby scoots down to the bottom of the bed and may turn around. You can try putting a rolled up towel across the bed so it raises her knees. Roll the towel very tightly and use tape to keep it from unrolling. Several commercially available wedges and slings (see resource list) keep your baby from sliding.

If your baby already accepts her familiar bed, you may want to raise the bed a little at a time and give your baby a few days to get used to the change. On the other hand, if she already hates her bed, you may be better off changing it a lot so she doesn't recognize that you are putting her in that horrible bed.

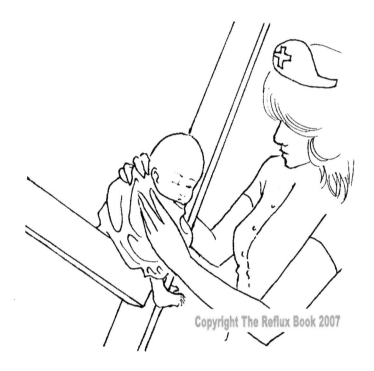

Copyright The Reflux Book 2007

Illustration 7: A slant board from the 1950s.

The original sleeping device used by hospitals was just a long board wrapped with towels that leaned against a wall. It had a peg sticking up out of it and the baby was placed face down on the board straddling the peg. The baby was kept in this position by tying her on with bandages or strips of fabric. We have come a long way!

To raise one end of the crib a few inches, you can buy bed lifts from any bedding store. Some parents have bolted longer legs to the crib or used a saw to cut off the legs toward the foot of the crib. It is sometimes possible to raise the head of the crib by resting it on a chair or small coffee table.

When you raise one end, the crib may become unstable and prone to tipping over. Test the stability by rocking the crib. Remember that your baby will soon be standing in the crib and trying to climb out. It should also be stable enough that a sibling or dog can't tip the crib over.

Some parents raise one end of the mattress rather than tilt the whole crib frame. If you stuff pillows under the mattress, the surface may be too squishy and bouncy and it may be possible for your baby to slip down under the mattress and suffocate.

You can raise the mattress and keep it stiff by inserting a piece of plywood at an angle to make a second crib bottom. The plywood should be exactly as wide as the crib and about 10-15" longer. It needs to fit very snugly. Elevating the head of the bed means that your baby can fall out easier when she learns to stand up unless you use a crib lid/tent. Again, this type of homemade solution is not advocated by the American Academy of Pediatrics.

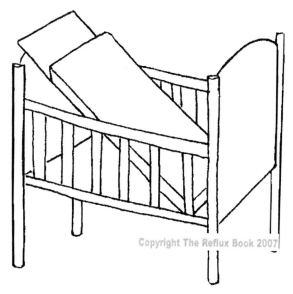

Illustration 8: *A crib with a second, tilted floor added*

Never assemble a crib with one end lower than the other unless the instructions that come with the crib say this is safe. It could fall apart.

Hammock

A reflux hammock (Amby Baby) is a special device that looks like an infant swing and keeps a baby positioned at an incline. It is used instead of a bed. The special construction keeps the baby from slipping down or turning on her tummy.

The US Consumer Product Safety Commission has recalled a different style of hammock that hangs inside a crib frame. The CPSC has also banned the use of plain string hammocks because babies have suffocated in them or managed to put their heads over the edge.

Co Sleeping

Many parents of babies with reflux find that the only way they can get any sleep is to keep the baby with them at night. Be extremely careful if you sleep deeply. Never put your baby between mom and dad. Studies show that the baby is much safer on mom's side of the bed as mothers tend to sleep less deeply and seldom roll over on their babies. Never drink or use medications that make you sleepy if you take your baby to bed with you. Never sleep with your baby on the couch because the squishy cushions can suffocate your baby if she rolls over. Never bring your baby into a waterbed.

A commercially made co-sleeper is a three-sided bassinet that fastens to the parents' bed. It keeps baby safe on her own sleep surface while keeping her close to you.

Be sure to also read the chapter called, Sleep or Lack Thereof .

Spoiling the Baby

You may have been told that you are spoiling the baby by holding her all day and she will never be able to sooth herself or play independently. Someone may have told you that rocking your baby to sleep and sleeping with her at night will make her clingy and dependent as a toddler and beyond. In addition, there are "baby trainers" who instruct parents on how to train the baby to eat, sleep and behave.

Unfortunately, baby training does not work when an infant or child is experiencing chronic pain and discomfort. When you know your baby is feeling better or has outgrown the reflux, you may need to help her learn self-soothing and greater independence, especially for sleeping. You will know when she is ready.

I nursed my daughter to sleep until she was 33 months old. She often woke at night and wanted to nurse once or twice. Doctors and relatives told me on more than one occasion that I was creating a sleeping problem by nursing her on demand. They implied that I would never be able to get her out of my bed. It wasn't until she was on a high dose of medication that she started sleeping through the night and became less dependent on the nursing. I was able to wean her pretty easily because I wasn't the "medicine" anymore. As she got older, she taught herself how to go to sleep and became very attached to her toddler bed. We never had to train her to go to sleep or bribe her. The medication took care of the underlying problem and allowed her to move forward. I never let her feel that she was abandoned when she wasn't feeling well. I think this really helped in the long run.

Notes:

6 FEEDING TIPS

You may have already noticed that feeding a baby with reflux is challenging. It may seem like your baby doesn't like to eat or has no appetite. It may take a great deal of trial and error to find a successful diet. This chapter is about how to feed your baby and the next chapter will give you information about choosing foods

A baby with significant reflux may experience pain and discomfort with each feeding. This chapter will show you unusual feeding patterns that can sometimes arise in babies with reflux. It will also give you a long list of parent-tested tricks to help feedings be more comfortable.

There are a wide variety of feeding problems in babies with reflux. The feeding strategies that work for one baby won't always work for other babies. Remember, the best feeding option for you and your baby is the one that provides digestive comfort for your baby.

The ultimate goal is to help your baby get adequate nutrition and develop normal eating patterns. Eventually, you want her to eat when she is hungry, and not eat when she isn't. You want her to eventually eat most of the foods that other children her age eat in the appropriate quantities so that she can maintain a healthy weight. Most parents also want their children to be open to trying new food experiences.

One of the reasons that we now pay more attention to reflux is that researchers have learned that poor nutrition can have more serious health affects than we realized. Growth charts were not in common use in the 1960s and were revised in the 1990s to put more emphasis on poor growth. There are several special growth charts including one for premature babies and even one for Asian babies who tend to be a bit small.

Growth charts are a standard way of monitoring growth but they need to be balanced with common sense. If the baby's parents are very small and the baby starts small, there is no reason to expect she should be in the middle of the chart. The doctor will watch weight, length and head circumference for trends on the chart that indicate a worrisome pattern could be developing.

Feeding issues for older children are discussed in a separate chapter in the Advanced Section of this book. Advanced topics addressing severe feeding problems are also in that chapter.

Reflux Feeding Patterns

Happy Spitter

The Happy Spitter eats with ease, then promptly urps or burps, smiling as the vomit dribbles down her chin. She doesn't experience any pain or discomfort from eating or spitting. She will grow just fine if she is able to keep down enough food or if you re-feed after she has vomited. Doctors are usually not concerned about this pattern and refer to it as a "laundry problem" rather than a "medical problem."

Happy spitters don't normally need any medical treatment. Tricks such as feeding her half as much and twice as often, keeping her upright for 30 minutes after meals and adequate burping can cut the spitting a bit and help keep those adorable outfits from smelling like curdled milk.

Fussing and Crying During Feeding

Does your baby fuss, cry and pull away from the breast or bottle? Does it feel like you are wrestling your baby and trying to find a comfortable position for both you and your baby? Some babies begin nursing or drinking eagerly then pull away and fuss/protest for the rest of the feeding. Babies who cry and fuss during feeding are probably experiencing pain with eating. Her tummy wants food but her throat and esophagus can't handle the pain. No wonder she acts confused and agitated during a meal.

My daughter would aggressively attack the bottle for a few seconds, and then suddenly stop with a cry. This pattern escalated until she didn't really want the bottle, only taking it once the hunger pain was worse than the reflux pain.

Fussing and Crying After Feeding

On the other hand, your baby may finish her meal without a whimper but then cries of pain may follow each meal.

Other babies do not experience pain until long after a meal has occurred. As the food is digested, it is mixing with acid. Wet burps or spit-ups that occur immediately after the meal may not hurt much. The later burps and urps become more acidic and may hurt more.

Poor Appetite or Small Stomach

Some parents report that their fussy babies do not signal the need to eat. Even if they skipped a feeding, it would not make a great deal of difference in comfort.

A variation of this is the baby who will willingly eats, but only a tiny amount at each meal and it may take an hour to get her to drink two ounces. She acts like her stomach is extra small and she won't eat as much or as fast as most babies.

Overeating

Some babies are greedy eaters. They eat too much, too fast and guzzle too much air in the process. Their little tummies can't handle so much food and this provokes reflux episodes. Often these babies go from hunger to 'starving' in just a few short minutes. Your baby might demand to be fed and get frantic if you take too long getting ready. She may eat a full meal in a matter of minutes and will get mad if you try to burp her. She eats so fast that her stomach is stretched and bloated before her brain realizes she is no longer hungry and tells her to stop eating.

Some babies have a circular pattern of over-eating and crying. Here is a typical pattern - your baby cries from hunger but finds that the bottle or breast adds a different kind of pain since the liquid is now burning her throat and esophagus. She may alternate between fussing and eating, ingesting quite a bit of air in the process. Now her stomach is full to the point that there is pain and discomfort from ingested air and bloating. The crying is from pain and bloating, not from hunger. Despite the fact that her stomach is full, she may want to drink in an effort to wash away the bad taste in her mouth. However, the additional liquid leads to more crying from bloating. Now over an hour has passed and it is hard to tell what to do. She seems like she wants to drink some more but she has been eating for over an hour. She won't stop crying and she is arching and kicking as you try every way to position her and soothe her. It may seem like she is unhappy whether her stomach is full or empty. No wonder you are worn out!

Comfort Eater

The comfort eater wants to eat and drink 24/7. She may want to nurse constantly whether awake or asleep to sooth the burning in her throat. She may want to eat frequent small meals so her stomach doesn't get too full, causing bloating and pain. Often, comfort eaters grow rapidly and may even be overweight. Older children who are comfort eaters may graze all day, seldom eating a real meal.

> *I feel like I am running a 24 hour diner...he wants to eat all day and all night. Needless to say, he is gaining weight very rapidly. The doctor says his weight and frequent feedings will normalize when he is out of pain.*

Dream Feeding

A dream feeder is an infant who is experiencing a great deal of pain from eating. She can turn off the pain by eating while asleep. You may find that you wait for your baby to go to sleep to initiate feeding. Other times, your baby protests and cries during a meal and falls into an exhausted sleep. Then you can begin the feeding.

Dream feeding works well with young infants because they are likely to sleep for long hours. Older babies who prefer dream feeding may need to be fed all night after a day of feeding refusal. Parents find that they are desperate for their dream feeders to go to sleep so they can feed them and get enough calories in. A better strategy would be to get the reflux under control so dream feeding isn't needed.

> *If we had not fed our daughter through the night, we would have had to place her on a feeding tube, which has a far greater negative effect on future feeding habits than dream feeding.*

As you work toward decreasing pain, dream feeding may offer a short-term feeding solution. It isn't a great long-term solution because babies who dream feed won't learn normal eating patterns. They don't get rid of their fears so they won't learn that food is good and satisfies hunger.

Feeding Aversion

A baby who experiences pain with each feeding may decide that she is going to "fix" the problem by not eating.

You may want to keep track of the amount she drinks and the number of wet diapers and report this information to the doctor. Babies dehydrate very quickly so it is important to have your baby evaluated by a doctor if you suspect she has significantly reduced the amount she is eating.

A feeding strike means that your baby is refusing all food and drink. She needs to be seen by a doctor today. It may be necessary to go to the emergency room if the doctor is not available.

The doctor will evaluate your baby to consider if an illness such as an ear infection or thrush is causing loss of appetite or if pain from reflux is causing a feeding strike.

She just clamped her little mouth shut and refused to take my breast all day. My mom tried giving her a bottle of formula and we even tried oral hydration drink. We were desperate. My mom held her while I worked to get a few drops of expressed breast milk into her mouth with a medicine dropper. It took an hour to get one ounce in. I finally called the pediatrician and he said to bring her right in. He said she was dehydrated and that we needed to get the reflux under control right away.

When a baby associates feeding with pain, just the sight of the bottle or breast is enough to cause distress.

Our doctor wanted to see what happened when I fed her. Just as soon as I showed my baby the bottle, she started shrieking. Our doctor said she didn't believe it until she saw it with her own eyes.

If your baby seems to be headed toward a feeding strike, you need to contact her doctor and you may want to read the Advanced Feeding chapter in the Advanced Section of this book.

Failure-to-Thrive

In some cases, a baby with reflux disease will eat so little or vomit such large quantities that growth slows down. In older children, picky eating and restricted diets may lead to poor nutrition and growth.

The term *Failure-to-Thrive* was once used to imply that a child was neglected or abused, missing developmental milestones and not growing as much as expected. This loaded term has gradually lost its original connotation. Now it is commonly used just to mean *poor weight gain or growth.*

Failure-to-thrive is a medical condition that needs to be monitored closely by the physician. This is especially vital in the first six months. In rare cases, a baby may need to be hospitalized for severe failure to thrive.

You may need to bring your baby to the doctor for frequent check-ups and weight checks. Your doctor may measure your baby's head circumference and height with each weight check. The doctor may also measure mom and dad's height and ask about their growth as infants. He may observe whether mom and dad have big bones or small bones by measuring the wrists.

> *My son started throwing up when he was 10 days old. He was never hungry. It took him two hours to finish 2 ounces of formula. Needless to say, he grew very slowly, but he stayed on the weight chart somehow. We thought he was just small because I am 5 ft tall with size 4 rings. But his daddy is over 6 foot and has very large bones so the pediatrician said our son really should be bigger than he is.*

Having a baby who is either underweight or a poor eater can be very difficult emotionally. Having a baby who is both can be very traumatic. It is hard to remember that you are a good mother when you can't even feed your own baby enough to keep her from starving. It can be challenging to keep your perspective in the face of this.

> *"Failure-to-Thrive." When my pediatrician uttered those words, I was reduced to tears. I was scared. I was angry. I was doing more than was humanly possible for my daughter, yet she wasn't thriving!?! I was hurt. It kind of struck at what it is to be a mother, I wasn't a good nurturer. I thought the "diagnosis" was heartless and almost changed pediatricians. For a while, it really affected my ability to work with him to help my daughter.*

Tips for Feeding Your Baby

Small, Frequent Feeding

It may be helpful to feed your baby small, frequent meals so that she is never too full and never too hungry. While baby books may tell you that it is important to get baby on a schedule and wait 3-4 hours between feeding, that advice may not apply to a baby with reflux. By letting her nibble a bit here, a bit there, she is putting less pressure on her stomach and learning to regulate her intake. She can sense when she needs to eat and start to signal you when she needs more.

Breastfeeding Tips

The first step to success is positioning your baby on the breast to ensure a good latch on. This will minimize air intake with feedings and reduce digestive discomfort from trapped air in the stomach.

It may be necessary to keep your baby as upright as possible while nursing. Some moms can lie down in a semi reclined position (with the baby face down on their breast) to increase comfort and decrease reflux episodes. Also, try nursing while standing up or with your baby in a sling.

Offering only one breast at each feeding is a common strategy for babies with reflux. This prevents the baby from overfilling her stomach.

Another common cause of choking, gagging or refusing the breast is an overactive letdown. This can be alleviated by pumping for a few seconds and then resuming nursing.

Remember, it takes two to tango. You and your baby need to work together to make nursing successful. Often, too much blame is placed on the mother for nursing failure. However, the baby may not be doing her part correctly. A lactation specialist or a La Leche leader may be able to assist you with specific difficulties and may be able to see if the baby is having problems nursing.

Your baby needs to have a coordinated suck and a good seal on the nipple to stimulate the milk and take in nourishment.

A baby who is in pain may fight the breast. A lactation consultant may be able to judge whether your baby appears to be in pain while nursing and whether reflux or some other illness is causing the pain.

Nursing for too short of a time can cause problems that increase reflux. Babies require the right proportion of foremilk (expressed at the beginning of a nursing session) and hind milk (from deeper in the breast). If your baby only gets the foremilk, which is high in lactose and low fat and doesn't get the high fat, high calorie hind milk, it can result in weight issues, fussiness and gassy, smelly bowel movements.

La Leche League has a booklet called Breastfeeding Your Baby with Reflux that was written by PAGER board member, Laura Barmby. This 17-page booklet has many more practical ideas.

Change Nighttime Feeding

The other babies (you know - the ones without reflux) in your new moms group may have learned to eat enough during the day that they sleep peacefully all night. Your baby may be eating less during the day so that night feedings are necessary to get caught up on calories. You may have heard others tell you that she is too old to be waking up at night and you need to "teach" her to stop bothering you at night. When she is able to eat a bigger meal without distress, you can certainly encourage her to sleep at that point. Perhaps you can eliminate one night feeding at a time until she is able to sleep all night.

It helps to be aware that some babies with reflux sleep much better when their tummies are empty because they have fewer reflux episodes when there is nothing in their stomachs. Some babies wake from hunger and some wake from reflux. Careful observation may help you figure out why your baby is waking. Hunger and reflux look alike.

> I had always heard that babies sleep better and longer on a full stomach so we always put her to sleep shortly after her last bottle. One night, we were out doing errands and she fell asleep without a bottle. I was shocked that she slept so much better. For the next several nights, we drove in circles around the neighborhood without her bottle till she was sound asleep. It worked.

Some babies are so underweight that the pediatrician may want you to add night feedings rather than subtract them.

Use Distraction

Some babies eat better when they are not thinking about eating. For some children, this means feeding in a quiet room when they are sleepy or half-asleep. Your baby may like to be wrapped securely in a blanket to minimize movement and help her relax. You may have seen the nurse swaddle your baby in the hospital.

For some children, distraction means keeping them entertained so they don't notice they are eating. You have better luck feeding these babies at the mall than in a quiet room. If they are doing something fun, you can sneak food into their mouths.

> *When our son was born, I banished the TV from the house. But when our daughter was eating so poorly that she couldn't gain weight, we got it back out. I'd place her in her highchair and sprinkle some Cheerios over the tray. She'd go into that hypnotic gaze that kids do in front of a TV and the Cheerios would disappear. The weight went back on. Now I have a healthy 4 year old who is an adventurous eater and watches at most 2 hours of TV a week. So even a mom who doesn't think that TV is worthwhile for kids, found TV to be a lifesaver for her GERD child. Just don't tell grandma!*

Minimize Air Intake with Feeding

Regardless of whether you are nursing or bottle feeding, it is important to ensure a good latch so that baby's lips are sealed around the bottle or breast. You can test whether she has a good seal by gently pulling back the nipple to see if she is able to keep her mouth around the bottle. If the bottle comes out of her mouth easily or she is a noisy eater, she may not have a good latch and seal.

A good seal will decrease the intake of air with each suck minimizing bloating and discomfort. Your baby may think she is full when she is just full of air. Crying can also increase air intake. Frequent burping may be necessary to release the trapped air.

Some types of baby bottles are designed to decrease air intake during drinking. If it looks like your baby has a good seal on the bottle and she is still burping or passing a lot of gas, you may want to try a different bottle or nipple. Many parents report that special bottles help a lot.

My gastroenterologist says: Do the sniff test. If she is swallowing air, the gas she passes won't stink. If she is eating food that doesn't agree with her, the gas, and sometimes the burps, will be smelly!

Burp Thoroughly

When your baby has reflux, it is even more important to burp her thoroughly. The goal is to get all the air out of her tummy very soon after she finishes eating. Every burp may bring up a bit of milk, but burps that come up later are bound to bring up more acid as well as milk.

If your baby is difficult to burp, experiment with different methods. Ask friends, neighbors and grandma for their tricks.

Trying to burp my daughter by patting her on the back was useless. The only thing we found that worked was to sit her upright in her car seat for ten minutes and let the bubbles all float to the top of her stomach. When she started to squirm and thrust her chin out, we would lift her by her armpits and let her feet dangle. She burped loud enough to impress her older brother!

Somebody from another country showed me how they burp babies. He held my baby and did a slow deep knee bend. Then he stood up suddenly and she burped. He called it "elevator ride."

Rate and Flow

It may be important to adjust the rate and flow of the milk supply. If the milk is coming out too fast, your baby may take giant gulps of milk and she will swallow too much air at the same time. If the rate is too slow, she may get too tired and give up on eating before she is full.

If you are breast-feeding, the letdown can sometimes produce a gush of milk and cause choking and gasping. You can use a pump, press a washcloth over your breast or use nipple shields until the letdown is over.

The nipple on a bottle may be switched to regulate the rate and flow of milk. Some parents report that they have tried several types of bottles and nipples before finding one that is just right for their little one. Dr. Brown's Bottles, angled bottles and Haberman Feeders, are popular.

If your baby likes to keep sucking until she over-fills her tummy, you can try switching to a very slow nipple when she is almost done with her bottle. This means she can suck that last ounce slower and satisfy her need to keep sucking. The Controlled Flow Baby Feeder is a bottle that lets you adjust the flow.

Thickening Formula and Breast Milk

One of the oldest treatments for reflux is to put cereal in the bottle to make the milk thicker and bounce less. Thickening is no longer as popular as it used to be but it works extremely well for some babies. One reason it may work is because it lets you give your baby a little bit less formula. For example, you can feed her five ounces instead of six, but she will still get enough calories. The smaller amount of liquid in the bottle means she doesn't over-fill her tummy.

There is some concern that cereal and other thickeners reduce the intake of nutrient rich formula or breast milk and adds too much "filler." The baby may gain weight from the extra calories but may have a decreased intake of vital nutrients because cereal is not nearly as nutritious as formula or breast milk. Some new studies show that thickened formula still supplies plenty of nutrition.

Some babies become constipated from rice cereal and other thickeners. There is also concern that adding food to an infant's diet too soon may increase the development of allergies.

A few babies gag and choke more on thickened feedings. Please monitor your baby closely if you choose to thicken. If thickened feeds decrease vomiting and help your baby to grow without the need for medication, this may be the best way to feed your baby.

Breast milk or formula may be thickened with rice cereal or another thickener such as oatmeal, barley or potato flakes. Read the labels carefully to make sure the thickener does not have any added ingredients such as soy.

Doctors often recommend adding one tablespoon of thickener such as rice cereal per ounce of liquid. Thickened liquids will be about as thick as tomato sauce or spaghetti sauce.

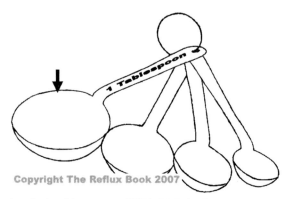

Illustration 9: *A tablespoon is USUALLY the largest spoon in the set. Check the markings to be sure. Sixteen tablespoons should equal a cup.*

It is difficult to thicken breast milk because the enzymes in the milk will break up the thickener and the milk thins out rapidly. It is best to thicken breast milk just before feeding or just thicken 1-2 ounces at a time. When your baby gets old enough to eat cereal, try giving her a few spoonfuls before nursing. A device called a soft feeder (by Medela) may help. It is a small bottle with a spoon instead of a nipple. The baby slurps the cereal instead of sucking it.

If adding cereal makes your baby gain too much weight, your doctor may recommend thickeners that don't have any calories. There are many brands of commercial thickeners on the market; ThickIt, Simply Thick, ThickenUp, Hydra Aid, Thick & Easy, Nutra Thick (has vitamins), Ready Care, Imperial, Thicken Right, Quick Thick and Thick Set.

If the doctor recommends thickening the bottle, it is best to purchase nipples that have an X or Y-shaped opening. Parents used to cut their own bottle nipples, but it is difficult to get them the same every time and your baby may end up with an overly fast flow one bottle and a slow flow for the next bottle.

Nipples for thick liquids are easily available and you should only cut your own in a pinch. To do this, take a clean pencil and insert the eraser end into the nipple. Use a very sharp knife or razor blade and cut downward using the eraser as a miniature cutting board. Some doctors recommend that you heat up a safety pin and use it to melt a larger hole in nipple.

Whether you use pre-cut nipples or cut your own, be very careful to get the nipples clean and sterilize them. The cuts can hold bacteria.

Learn to Read Your Baby's Hunger Cues

If your baby has discomfort from reflux, she may act like she is hungry. For some people, the pain of reflux feels a lot like hunger pains. And for some people, eating a little bit can help wash the acid back down into the stomach.

It may take some very careful observation on your part to tell when she is hungry and when she needs just a slurp or two to wash down the acid. She may think she needs a whole meal but if you just fed her recently and she eats again, she may become overly full and cause more reflux. She may be confused about whether she is hungry or experiencing esophageal pain and the cues she gives you may confuse you.

If she waits too long between feedings, she may be frantic and suck air in her effort to eat quickly and relieve the pain of hunger. She may be inclined to over-feed and get too full. It may help to start feeding her as soon as she acts hungry and not wait till she is desperate.

You need to work with her and read her signals - is she rooting for your breast or making a little fussing sound? She may be communicating to you that she is ready for a little snack. Remember, she said "little snack," not "three course meal!"

If you try to get her to finish the last few ounces in her bottle or take the other breast, she may eat more than her stomach needs now. See if you can start to tell when she is just full enough, but not too full. Maybe she is enjoying the closeness and keeps feeding because she wants to prolong the cuddling. You can see that she is sucking much slower and letting some dribble out. Or maybe she just wants to keep sucking slowly but isn't hungry anymore.

Positioning During and After Meals

Most babies with reflux do better if they are held upright while feeding. Finding the right position may feel very awkward for both of you. Ask a nurse or lactation specialist to help you find a comfortable position that allows your baby to be upright.

It may help to keep her legs straight so there is less pressure on her stomach. Curling her up into a little ball may place pressure on her stomach and literally squeeze the food right out. The result may be vomiting of her entire meal.

Part of what makes feeding enjoyable is the cuddling. She needs to be close to you so she can see you and feel the warmth of your body. Even if it hurts to eat, it may comfort her to know that you are there for her.

After a meal, your baby may need to be held in an upright position for up to 30 minutes to allow her to digest her meal and minimize vomiting. See the Home Care and Positioning Chapter for more information and cautions.

Manage Pain

Feeding an infant or child who is in pain from eating will lead to a great deal of frustration for all. A baby or child who experiences pain every time food goes down her throat will believe that eating equals pain. Eventually, this painful experience will be avoided at all costs. After all, we all work hard to avoid painful experiences, don't we?

A special diet, and perhaps medication will be necessary to lessen the pain and allow feeding to progress. It may take a great deal of time and positive experience to make feeding a safe and even pleasurable experience.

Watch for Food Allergies and Intolerances

It is possible for a baby or child to be allergic/intolerant to almost any food. Do-it-yourself reaction/allergy detective work is difficult and should only be done with your doctor's help. It can be especially hard to spot a food reaction if your child has regular reflux PLUS several food reactions. The diet is hard work and disruptive for the whole family.

Foods that cause allergies can cause an immediate or a delayed response. Delayed or slow responses are particularly difficult to tease out. They can take days to show up and a week or more to clear up once the food is removed.

The most common food allergies are milk, fish, shellfish, nuts, peanuts, wheat, soy and eggs.

The parents who seem to have the best luck figuring out food reactions come from families with a strong history of asthma, allergies, hay fever, eczema and food sensitivities.

> *Because of our experiences with our older son, my wife and I chose not to introduce solids until 6 months. It was well after a year when we started to introduce wheat, egg whites, corn, tomato, as well as dairy and soy. Papaya was an early hit, and that is good for digestion.*

Doctors and parents say that the following clues are useful to spot food reactions:

Spitting-up, vomiting or tummy aches after eating certain foods or ingredients

If your baby refuses certain foods

Skin rashes, patches of dry skin, eczema or hives (look like mosquito bites)

Rashes that develop after food has touched the skin

Areas of the body swell and look puffy, especially the lips or eyes

Wheezing or asthma symptoms after eating

Frequent runny noses that last longer than a cold

Bouts of constipation or diarrhea, especially if they alternate

Dark circles under the eyes or creases under the eyes

Ears turn bright red after eating

If your baby has a glassy look to her eyes or just stares without really paying attention to what is going on around her

If your child's reflux improves after switching to a new formula and then symptoms return after 1-2 weeks

Predigested / hydrolysate / hypoallergenic formulas are tolerated somewhat better than normal formulas

Smelly burps and gas

Bloody stools

Delay the Introduction of Foods

It is hard to say when your little one should start eating more than formula or breast milk. Many pediatricians recommend beginning foods between 4-6 months. You may find that your baby is ready to eat and eager to try new tastes and flavors. If your baby is clamping her mouth shut or looks uncomfortable during or after a meal, she may be telling you that she is not ready. It may be necessary to delay the introduction of solid foods such as baby food from a jar or mashed table foods.

There are several reasons why your baby may not be ready for foods. Some of the baby foods may be high in acid (fruits) causing a burning sensation on an irritated esophagus. If your baby isn't ready to swallow textures, the food will cause choking and coughing. Feeding skill development may be delayed if there has been an interruption in feeding due to an illness, food refusal or a feeding tube.

Your baby with reflux may just be cautious about trying new textures or flavors – especially if formula or breast milk feedings were difficult. She may be a little concerned about the spoon and bib after just starting to feel "safe" about drinking from a bottle.

> *My oldest son (without acid reflux) ate from a spoon at exactly 4 months of age. He would cry if I didn't shovel it in fast enough! My second son had severe reflux and we were lucky to get him to take a bottle, much less baby food from a spoon. Feeding was not pleasurable to him and he needed to stay with bottle-feeding a lot longer. There was no way I was going to play around with his feeding and add something new. We were both recovering from the work of feeding him while he was in pain. I had to introduce foods a lot more slowly and it took him a long time to think that food was "safe" let alone "fun."*

Make Food Fun

Your baby is getting all her nutrition from breast milk or formula so solid foods are not vital to nutrition. But playing with foods is one way that babies learn other skills. When she picks up tiny bits of food, she is using the muscles in her fingers and learning to focus her eyes carefully. And when she holds the bits of food over the floor and lets go of them, she learns that they fall. And then her parents make funny faces and pick them up. When little bits find their way into her mouth, she learns about salty and sweet. When she slobbers on a cookie, she learns that she can use it to draw on the table. When she plays with meat, she learns that the dog will sit right at her feet and wag his tail – he might even stand up and beg. When she puts her hand in ice cream, she learns about cold. When she sits at the table with other children and grown ups she learns to be sociable – for a few minutes.

Treat Feeding Problems Early

If your baby has a lot of trouble with foods, get help early. Despite medical treatment and home care, reflux can sometimes lead to feeding refusal and picky eating. Consulting a professional early may help get her back on track quicker.

Your baby's sensory system may be making it hard for her to eat. The sensory system (touch, taste, smell) has a huge impact on eating. While a particular food may taste fine or feel normal on your tongue, it may taste and feel awful to someone with a sensory problem.

The sensory system may over-react or it may under-react. For instance, a child may have a hyperactive gag reflex. Every time a textured food touches the back of the mouth, a strong gag reflex is activated. These children react quickly, and too strongly.

A child who avoids putting toys in her mouth and doesn't like new tastes and textures may have an overly active sensory system. This child may appear upset or agitated if someone touches around or in the mouth or even the cheeks and chin. To avoid stimulating an over active sensory system, a child may insist on a liquid diet or pureed foods. She may want a very bland diet and become upset if foods other than the "safe" foods are introduced. Attempts to touch the mouth or put textured food in her mouth will often result in crying, avoidance, choking and vomiting.

Some children have the opposite problem – they react too slowly. Food may be in all the wrong places and start to go down the wrong tube. Choking can occur if the sensory system does not signal the brain fast enough to deal with the bite of food. He may have trouble with solids because he doesn't seem to realize that they should be chewed (or gummed) before they are swallowed.

It just won't work to ignore the problem and force your baby to eat. It is a process, involving breaking old habits, building trust in eating and associating feeding with pleasure. This may take some hard work and time. In severe cases, a feeding therapist or feeding team may be needed.

Often, a speech therapist or an occupational therapist may be consulted to evaluate the nature of the sensory problem and offer treatment to normalize the sensory processing system.

> *My son has had reflux since birth. He refused solids. In fact, he would gag and throw up if we gave him anything thicker than baby food even at eight months old. He had a feeding evaluation and it was determined that he has what is called, "Sensory Integration Disorder." His therapist told me that it is common in children with reflux. It means that their body has a hard time accepting things with texture. It also shows up in some kids as not liking things on their feet or hands – he thought touching food was gross. He has been going to therapy for 2 months now and we have seen a big improvement.*

Dealing with Feeding Advice and Myths

You may get a lot of advice from others about when to start spoon-feeding and what to feed first. Some will warn you that there is a critical time to begin feeding or it will be difficult for your baby to learn to eat. Others will tell you that she needs to be exposed to all textures, flavors and food groups or she will not eat a variety of foods later on.

> *I always felt like friends and relatives were judging me. We all know spoiling your child is parenting sin #1 and giving in to a picky eater is parenting sin #2.*

Most parents firmly believe the myth that food avoidance is a form of misbehaving. They do not realize that a baby who avoids food is almost certainly doing so for a very logical reason. A toddler may go through a temporary stage of refusing to do what you want because it is her job to test her independence and see how you react. But babies don't do this.

Most parents believe that all children will eat if you let them get hungry enough. This is simply not true. Some children have medical problems that interfere with their appetite and a fair number of children with reflux are afraid to eat because it causes pain. Eating is not purely instinctive – it is very complex and some babies need extra time or help.
You may feel offended by feeding advice from others because it seems like a reflection of your parenting. But the reality is: there are no rules for feeding a baby with reflux and there is no magical "right" way.

You may get some wonderful ideas from parents of other children who have similar reflux symptoms, but they may not all work for you. Pick and choose what to try. It is also very helpful to learn from parents whose children have been in feeding programs.

I've been through feeding hell with my daughter...and made it to the other side. She had flared up horribly when we introduced solids at 6 months and it took forever to get the fire out. We went on medication and finally the screaming stopped. But she wouldn't eat. She wouldn't even go into the kitchen where I had the high chair. She'd scream bloody murder. She got her nutrition at night, nursing every hour on the hour while she slept. I finally called the pediatric gastroenterologist and his nurse gave me memorable advice: relax and enjoy your baby. I hung up in disgust.

What should be a pleasurable experience can be made quite miserable...it got me thinking about what I was doing to my daughter. I was so desperate for her to eat that I always had a baggie full of Cheerios in my pocket. We'd be out on a walk and I would be stuffing them into her face rather then allowing her to enjoy herself. I would try to distract her with videos and stuff food into her face.

I decided to let her be in control of her eating. If she wanted to eat, fine. If not, well she could nurse eight times at night. I took all the pressure off of her. Now this wasn't easy. She was failure to thrive, below the lowest line on the growth chart but she wasn't falling further behind. I took the nurse's advice and willed myself to relax and enjoy my baby. This was the most difficult thing I have ever done.

A couple of weeks later she wanted to come into the kitchen, but not into the high chair. Then the high chair, but not eating. Finally, nibbling. She gained confidence that eating was no longer painful. And she gained confidence that I wouldn't be "encouraging" her to eat. For the past year, she has been an awesome eater. She loves to eat! She tried EVERYTHING-not one hint of fussy toddler eating with her. She eats with such gusto and enjoyment!

Now none of this would have worked if her reflux wasn't under super control. That's the cornerstone. And even when the pain behavior stops, it can take weeks for the esophagus to totally heal. But the "technique" that worked for me was really listening to my baby - letting her tell me when she was ready. I discovered that one of her big hang-ups was that she didn't want to wear a bib. I accepted the mess and she responded by eating better. I discovered that she didn't want baby food from a jar-she wanted finger foods that she could feed herself. But these were things that I couldn't hear until I let go of my anxiety.

Notes:

7 WHAT TO FEED YOUR BABY

Some parents say that feeding their baby with reflux is the most challenging thing they have ever done. You may find that you are doing a great deal of experimenting to find the right food for your baby. For mild reflux, a careful diet combined with feeding techniques may be the only medical treatment your baby needs.

Your baby's doctor is the best source of advice for what to feed your baby. All diet changes should be made with supervision from the pediatrician. The best food for your baby is the food that causes the least amount of distress to her digestive system. You and the pediatrician will have to work together to figure out which foods are best for your baby.

Breast is Best

With rare exceptions, breast milk is best for an infant with reflux. Breast milk digests faster than formula and fast digestion minimizes reflux. Babies with reflux are often prone to catching every illness that runs through the neighborhood. Breast milk boosts your baby's immune system and provides protection from illnesses that formula can't match.

You may find that breastfeeding decreases your workload because it is available on demand and doesn't need to be prepared. An added benefit is that when you nurse, hormones that help you relax are released, a real bonus when you are dealing with a fussy baby all day.

In the past, it was believed that all babies with reflux needed to be on thickened formula and doctors discouraged mothers from breastfeeding. We now know that babies with reflux usually do better with breast milk.

Nursing Mother's Diet

There is some evidence that some babies with reflux feel less digestive distress if the mother eliminates foods that are most likely to cause food allergies: Milk, soy, tree nuts, peanuts, wheat and eggs.

Some mothers believe that eliminating other foods makes a definite difference for their babies. The typical foods they eliminate are broccoli, onions, garlic, cabbage, caffeine, spices, tomatoes, chocolate and alcoholic beverages.

If the baby has a known food allergy, the nursing mother will need to eliminate the food from her diet. When an allergy is suspected, a mother may choose to try a strict elimination diet for a few weeks before gradually adding one food at a time to determine which foods are not tolerated. Elimination diets should be supervised by your Internist, OB/GYN or Family Practitioner. Your baby is depending on you and you can't risk your own health.

Often it is very stressful to a nursing mother to eat a restricted diet since there isn't always time to read labels, shop carefully and prepare meals from scratch. In addition, it isn't always clear that eliminating foods from your diet has made a difference.

There is a great deal of controversy about the need to eliminate food groups from a nursing mother's diet. Many nursing mothers tell us that certain foods cause more spit-up and fussiness. Other mothers tell us removing all forms of dairy made a difference. It is important to talk with your doctor and even a nutritionist to ensure that both you and your baby get the nutrients you need.

> *I did try an elimination diet after the medication just didn't help a bit. After being on the diet for two weeks, I did notice that my son was a little better. I added back eggs and everything seemed OK. A week later my son was actually doing really well, so I decided to reintroduce soy. Immediately all of the symptoms came back - pulling off the breast, screaming, refusing to nurse and general fussiness and unexplained screaming periods. After only 2 days of eating soy products, it has taken a full week to get my son back to "normal." I feel like the elimination diet has picked up where the medicine failed.*

Maintaining Your Breast Milk Supply

The quality of the breast milk is affected by your diet and a healthy life-style. If your diet is severely limited because of a special diet or you are extremely stressed and sleepless, the quantity and quality of your milk may decrease. It is also important to stay hydrated to maintain your sup-ply.

> *My milk supply was drying up because I was trying to take care of the children and the household and the baby would not sleep at night. My lactation specialist told me to go to bed with the baby - as if I had the flu. My family was to wait on me, bring me food and drinks and let us both rest for 24-48 hours if possible. I had a pitcher of water by the bed and I kept the door of the bedroom closed the whole time. My milk supply increased tremendously and the baby actually slept a little better. Maybe she was hungry and my supply was not keeping up with her intake.*

If your milk supply is seriously low, ask a lactation consultant about using a Supplemental Nursing System for a short time. It is a device that lets you hang a small bag of formula around your neck with a very thin tube that drips formula into the baby's mouth as she nurses.

Some mothers feel very disappointed when they can't nurse or nurse as long as they had planned. Even with a supportive family, or household help, it can be exhausting to stay on a special diet, take care of a baby night and day and get the nutrients you need. Even if you can nurse for a little while, you are giving your baby important benefits. Maybe you can still nurse her once a day.

Deciding to Try Formula

If you have struggled with nursing for a while or chose not to nurse, bottle-feeding may be the right choice. In the end, seeing your baby thrive, regardless of the diet, is the sweetest sight.

If you want to try formula for a few days, you can still maintain your milk supply. Simply pump your milk at regular intervals during the day and freeze it. If you find that she is just as unhappy with the formula as the breast milk, you have the option of going back to nursing or staying with bottle-feeding. Or you can do both – a bottle for some feedings and mother nature for others.

I was so convinced my milk was bad for my baby that I switched to formula. Talk about jumping out of the frying pan into the fire! Now we are on the musical formula merry-go-round and he is much worse.

◆

I had already tried three formulas without success and the doctor suggested yet another formula. The difference was like night and day. He was less fussy right from the first bottle and has gotten progressively better with time. We are now vomit free except for the occasional spit up! He can eat 6 ounces at a time and last night he slept 9 hours! He is so tremendously different - just so happy! My husband and I are both so relieved.

The advantages of formula include: control over ingredients and elimination of possible allergens. An additional benefit of bottle-feeding is that feeding and night waking duties can be shared with another caretaker.

All of the infant formulas on the market claim different benefits and ingredients to promote growth and development. The bottom line is all formulas strive to achieve what breast milk does.

You and your doctor may have considered different formulas as a treatment since some babies seem to digest certain kinds of formula better than others. You may have noticed that some formulas are milk or soy based while others are lactose free, pre digested or hypoallergenic. Some infant formula is even thickened. There is no single formula that is perfect for all babies with reflux.

Finding the Right Formula

Parents and doctors may find that they need to try more than one formula before finding one that is a good match for the baby. Parents often need to monitor the baby and convey observations to the doctor about tolerance of the formula. Clues that a formula may not be a good match for your baby are: constipation, increased fussiness, vomiting, skin rash, blood in the stool or diaper rash.

The variety in infant formulas can be overwhelming. This list will help you understand why your doctor is making certain recommendations.

Formulas are grouped based on the amount and type of protein they contain.

All infant formulas sold in the United States are certified by the government to provide complete nutrition. Do not use cow's milk, goat's milk, soymilk or rice milk. These beverages lack important vitamins.

Milk Based: contains whole dairy proteins.
Lactose Free Formula: Milk based formula with no milk sugar.
AR: Milk based formula with added rice thickener.
Soy Based: Contains whole soy proteins.
Partly Hydrolyzed Formula with partly broken down proteins. Often marketed as "gentler."
Soy based with broken soy proteins
Whey based with broken milk proteins
Casein based with broken milk proteins
Extensively Hydrolyzed with well-broken proteins. Marketed as "hypoallergenic" but some babies still react.
Soy based with well broken soy proteins
Whey based with well broken milk proteins
Casein based with well broken milk proteins
Amino Acid / Elemental: No proteins or partial proteins at all. Lowest chance of allergic reactions although rare reactions do occur – usually reactions to the carbohydrates or sugars.

Babies with Milk Soy Protein Intolerance and some children with allergies react to proteins of any sort and must use amino acid formulas. Amino acids are the building blocks of proteins. When a person eats proteins, they are broken down into amino acids, which are then used to build new proteins like muscles.

Keep in mind that amino acid based formula is very expensive and should be used under the direction of a physician. Insurance may cover the cost, but many companies deny coverage for these expensive formulas. You can appeal the decision by writing letters or having your doctor write to your insurance company.

If your baby has some signs of allergy, the doctor may suggest trying a hydrolyzed formula for two weeks. Some doctors suggest an elemental formula for two weeks as a test.

Many parents report that their children react differently when they eat the ready-to-feed and powdered versions of the same formula. New research shows this is true, but nobody seems to understand why. Most babies tolerate the powder better, but your baby may like the ready-to feed version.

Practical Formula Hints

It is very important to measure formula accurately. Put the correct amount of water in the bottle first and then add the formula powder. If you put the powder in first, you won't get the water measured correctly.

Mix the formula exactly according to the directions on the can unless your doctor gives you other instructions. Your doctor may tell you to use a tiny bit more formula in each bottle – do not do this on your own. Your baby needs enough water to be able to metabolize the nutrients. If you make it too strong, it might not be good for her.

If you mix formula ahead of time and refrigerate it, the bubbles have a chance to float to the top and your baby will get less air in her tummy. You can bang the bottle on the counter gently to get the bubbles out.

AR formula clumps if you mix it with warm water. It contains starch and warm water will cook the starch into small clumps like dumplings. AR formula will not appear to be thick in the bottle. It only thickens when it interacts with stomach acid. It may not thicken if your baby is on acid-reducing medications.

Pay Close Attention to Germs in Food

Your baby already has a delicate digestive system. You do not want to accidentally feed her something contaminated with bacteria. If she is on an acid reducing medicine, this is particularly important because she might not have enough stomach acid to kill the bacteria.

Don't save food that touches your baby's lips. One hour is the safe limit to finish a bottle or a jar of food. If your baby only eats half a jar of food at a time, pour half into a small bowl or cup so that you won't contaminate the jar with saliva when you put the spoon in it. Watch out for bottles that roll under the couch and disappear for days. Keep the high chair and bottles very clean.

Be very cautious about traveling with pre-mixed bottles. They need to be kept very cold so they don't spoil. It is often safer to travel with a bottle of room temperature water and keep the powdered formula in a small container with a good seal.

Starting Solids

It is common for babies with reflux to start on rice cereal very early and wait a long time before trying other foods. Your baby is getting all her nutrition from breast milk or formula so solids are not necessary for nutrition. Ask your doctor when your gerdling should try solids. If you have a family history of allergies, it might be best to wait.

Most babies with reflux tolerate rice cereal and vegetables that are yellow or orange. If she happily tolerates these, the next thing to try is usually green vegetables, but many gerdlings just vomit them up. She may like fruits, but many babies with reflux can feel the acid in fruit and they will refuse to eat it. Bananas from a jar may be tolerated better than other fruit. Mashed bananas may be a bit harder to digest. The small red bananas from the gourmet section may be easier on her tummy. Because so many babies with reflux react badly to high protein foods, meats and eggs are often last on the list of things to try.

You may also need to wait for several months to try thicker foods or finger foods. Mixed textures – purees or liquids with lumps in them - can confuse your baby when she tries to swallow them.

It is helpful to introduce one new food at a time in small amounts and then wait about three days to see if you get a reaction. If you have a family history of food reactions, you may want to do three trials of the same food - give your baby a bit more of that same food on day three and then wait three more days. If you don't see any problems, feed a much larger quantity of the same food on day six and wait three more days to see if it causes any problems. Large quantities of some foods can cause constipation or diarrhea but you won't see this with just a few spoonfuls.

Notes:

8 MEDICATIONS

The chapter will provide an overview of the medications used to treat reflux disease and address common questions about how they work. The next chapter has information on how to actually get the medication into your baby successfully.

You will not see recommendations on the best medication or a dosing guide in this book because there is no best medicine or best dose that works for all children. That is for you and your doctor to determine.

It may be alarming to read the list of potential side effects of the medications in this chapter. Keep in mind that the vast majority of babies and children tolerate medication with no side effects at all. If side effects occur, they are usually mild and often go away after the body has adjusted to the medication. We have only listed the side effects that are fairly common. For a full list of side effects, consult your pharmacist or the Physician's Desk Reference at your local library. Some manufacturers have complete "prescribing information" on their web sites or inside the box of medication. This is the same as the package insert.

If you look at the official information sheet of any medication, you will see a very scary, very long list of side effects. Keep in mind that when a drug is being tested, any illness or symptom that occurs during the study is noted. If a child happens to have an ear infection (common) while he is in a study for a reflux medication, ear infections will be listed as a "side effect" of taking the medication. If you observe new symptoms or possible side effects from a medication, it is always best to consult with your doctor right away.

Over the past few decades, there have been many changes in the way children with reflux are medicated. Until the mid 1990s, the only medicines that were in common use were antacids and H2 blockers. These gave way to motility medications, which held great promise because they seemed to address the underlying cause of reflux in children, spontaneous lower esophageal sphincter or LES relaxation. Unfortunately, dangerous side effects were discovered with the most common motility medication and this whole class of medications is not used as often. In the 1990s a new class of medications, The Proton Pump Inhibitor or PPIs came into common use, first for adults, and later for children. They address the problem from a different angle – they suppress acid rather than improving the muscle tone. In the next decade or so, the trend will probably change again as newer, safer motility medications come on the market.

Naming Medicines

In the United States, medicines go by more than one name, which can make things confusing. The type of medication has a name such as H2 blocker. There may be several medications in each class. Each one had a chemical name – also called the generic name. We will use ranitidine as an example. It was the first H2 blocker on the market in the US.

The company that invents the chemical is the only company allowed to make that medicine for the first 17 years. They give the chemical a brand name such as Zantac, which is capitalized and is always the largest word on the box.

After 17 years, other companies can apply for permission to make their own version of the medicine in Zantac – a generic version of ranitidine. The original brand is usually the most expensive since the company that invented it spent a lot of money on testing the chemical and changing it until they got it right. So, when a generic version of the medicine becomes available, your insurance company may ask you to switch because the generic is cheaper.

Sometimes a medication is safe enough that the Food and Drug Administration will let manufacturers sell it directly to consumers without needing a prescription from a doctor. When a drug becomes available over-the-counter, the dosage may be the same or lower and the name may stay the same or be slightly different. Over-the-counter Zantac is known as Zantac 75 because it has 75 mg and the prescription version has 150 mg of medicine per dose. Ask your pharmacist what is most economical and practical for your child.

If the medicine has been on the market for more than 17 years, other companies may also start making an over-the-counter version of the generic medicine. If you pick up a store brand or generic brand of acid reducer, it may have exactly the same ingredient as the Zantac 75 sitting next to it on the shelf.

Medication manufacturers are always looking for new ways to market their products. We are now starting to see combinations of medications such as an H2 blocker that has been combined with an antacid. This is just like putting an anti-sneezing medicine and an anti-coughing medicine in the same bottle of cold medicine. It might be more convenient, but it is usually much more expensive.

Medications for the Treatment of Reflux Disease

H2 Blockers

Histamine 2 (H2) blockers work by reducing stomach acid production. H2 blockers interfere with the effect of one type of histamine and may offer a small amount of additional protection for those with food allergies.

Names

Brand Names (USA)	Generic Name/Main Ingredient
Axid	Nizatidine
Pepcid, Mylanta AR plus generics	Famotidine
Tagamet plus generics	Cimetidine
Zantac plus generics	Ranitidine

Practicalities

H2 blockers can be given "as needed" or daily for long-term relief of symptoms. Acid suppressors are generally given several times per day. They can be taken with food, but are more effective when taken on an empty stomach.

H2 blockers may interact with PPIs so they should be given at separate times of day. H2 blockers can affect the absorption of many other medicines, particularly those that need acid to be metabolized properly. It can also make some medicines absorb better so that the dose of the other medicine becomes too strong. Check with your pharmacist for a long list of interactions.

Some patients develop a tolerance to these medicines and they stop working. Switching brands may help. Some patients report rebound acid when these medicines are stopped abruptly. It may be better to wean off them.

Side Effects

Your child will probably not experience any side effects. H2 blockers can cause headaches, dizziness, nausea, constipation, diarrhea or stomach pain. Agitation and confusion have been reported as well as nightmares and night terrors. Rare side effects include breast swelling and the possibility of a higher incidence of pneumonia and gastrointestinal infections.

Use of H2 blockers could theoretically reduce absorption of iron, vitamin B-12 and calcium causing anemia, pernicious anemia or fragile bones. Long-term use of H2 blockers could theoretically unbalance the beneficial bacteria in the digestive system. In theory, the lack of stomach acid could make patients more susceptible to food poisoning from spoiled food.

Liquid Zantac contains alcohol. In addition, the chemical properties of H2 blockers prohibit the liver from processing alcohol correctly. Many parents don't like the idea of giving alcohol to a child. A melt-in-your-mouth-pill version exists. Ask your pharmacist.

Proton Pump Inhibitors

Proton Pump Inhibitors (PPIs) can almost completely eliminate stomach acid production. Most Proton Pump Inhibitors are time released meaning the medication is slowly released into the body, offering long-term relief of symptoms.

Names

Brand Names (USA)	Generic Name/Main Ingredient
AcipHex	Rebeprazole
Nexium	Esomeprazole
Prevacid	Lansoprazole
Prilosec and generics	Omeprazole
Protonix	Pantoprazole
Zegerid	Omprazole - immediate release
Kapidex	Dexlansoprasole – dual release

Practicalities

PPIs are often given once every 24 hours but some doctors recommend giving the medicine twice a day by splitting the dose.

PPIs are much more effective if given 30 minutes before a meal. The medicine needs to be in the blood stream when the foods hit your stomach to have the longest lasting effect. The timing can be just as important as the dosing.

New research shows that some children metabolize the medication very rapidly and may need several small doses rather than one large dose. Children age 1-10 often need doses that are larger for their weight than an adult would need. Your doctor can order something called pharmacokinetic testing to see if your child needs a higher dose or your doctor may just experiment with the doses to see if higher doses help.

At the moment, the PPIs are approved for teens and several are approved for younger children. Doctors are free to use these medicines on children of all ages but it is difficult to obtain dosing guidance for children who are not in the approved age range. Your doctor may need to call the manufacturer, a hospital pharmacist and consult several medical journals to decide on the dose.

Studies show that discontinuing PPIs abruptly may cause the stomach to make higher amounts of acid. This temporary rebound effect may be avoided by lowering the dose gradually rather than stopping suddenly.

Side Effects

Your child will probably not experience any side effects. PPIs can cause headaches, diarrhea, nausea, constipation and gas. Less common side effects include: dizziness, weakness, rash, vomiting, discolored bowel movements, stomach pain, and decreased hunger, changes in taste, muscle pain, joint pain, agitation, confusion, bad dreams, sleepiness, irritability, breast swelling and elevated liver enzymes. There is a higher incidence of pneumonia and gastrointestinal infections in patients on PPIs.

Use of PPIs can reduce absorption of iron and vitamin B 12 causing anemia or pernicious anemia.

Use of PPIs can interfere with calcium absorption in the stomach and they could theoretically affect the way in which old bone is replaced by new bone. Elderly patients using PPIs are at higher risk of breaking bones but nobody has studied this in children. Use of PPIs could theoretically unbalance the beneficial bacteria in the digestive system. In theory, the lack of stomach acid could make patients more susceptible to food poisoning from spoiled food.

Caution

Adult studies have shown that people of Asian descent may not be able to metabolize PPIs as well as others. They may need lower doses. There is some evidence that suggests newborns and young babies may not have the digestive enzymes to break down this type of medication.

PPIs may affect the absorption of other medicines, particularly those that need acid to be metabolized properly.

Antacids

Antacids are often used for adults to treat mild reflux and quickly neutralize acid that is already present in the stomach. Antacids work very quickly and come in many flavors and forms – look for tiny pills that can be swallowed, chewables and even sprinkles/powders.

Names

Brand Names (USA)	Main Ingredient
Tums	Calcium
Maalox	Aluminum and Magnesium

Children's Mylanta	Calcium
Rolaids	Calcium and Magnesium
Milk of Magnesia	Magnesium
Prelief	Calcium
Gaviscon	Aluminum and a foaming, barrier agent
Children's Pepto Bismol	Calcium. (Adult Pepto contains Bismuth subsalicylate, a chemical similar to aspirin and SHOULD NOT BE USED FOR CHILDREN)
Alka Seltzer	Contains aspirin and SHOULD NOT BE USED FOR CHILDREN

Practicalities

Antacids are typically used for patient with occasional bouts of reflux or used on days when a prescription medicine isn't enough. Antacids are inexpensive and don't require a prescription, but they should never be given to children unless recommended by the doctor.

The North American Society for Pediatric Gastroenterology, Hepatology and Nutrition (NASPGHN) does not recommend the use of antacids for long-term treatment. A doctor may suggest a short trial of antacids to see if reflux symptoms resolve and confirm a suspected diagnosis of reflux. A physician may prescribe them for occasional use.

Manufacturers of antacids may make several variations that have different ingredients. Read the labels carefully.

Side Effects

Your child may experience mild side effects. Antacids with magnesium may tend to cause diarrhea. Antacids with aluminum may tend to be constipating. None are safe to use at high doses for prolonged periods. There is some concern that antacids containing aluminum may inhibit calcium and zinc absorption.

Watch the artificial sugars in many antacids – some little tummies don't like them. Watch the real sugars that can cause cavities.

Physical Barriers

Physical barriers protect the esophagus and stomach from damage by providing a coating or barrier from acid exposure. The medication also floats on top of stomach contents and may provide a physical barrier to keep acid from backwashing into the esophagus.

This type of medication may be used to promote healing of the esophagus as well as to treat ulcers. A physical barrier can provide immediate relief from symptoms and very little is absorbed into the body.

There is little or no evidence that these medications reduce reflux symptoms or protect the esophagus from damage but many patients report symptom relief.

Names

Brand Names (USA)	Generic Name / Main Ingredient
Carafate	Sulcrafate
Gaviscon	Alginic Acid Slurry

Practicalities

Usually, this medication is given prior to a meal. The tablets easily dissolve in water.

Side Effects

Your child will probably not experience any side effects. Constipation is the only common side effect. Sulcrafate has properties similar to glue and rare reports exist of food balls (bezoars) which are somewhat similar to hairballs getting stuck in the stomach.

Caution

This type of medication may prevent the absorption of other medications so ask your doctor or pharmacist for assistance.

Motility Medications

Motility medications or Prokinetics move food through the GI tract more effectively and a bit faster by making the muscles work better. They can tighten the lower esophageal sphincter muscle. Motility drugs may be used for children with delayed emptying of the stomach and children suspected of aspirating. They are only effective for some children.

No prokinetic agent available in the United States and Canada, including metaclopramide and bethanechol, has been shown to be effective in the treatment of GERD in children. – NASPGHN

Names

Brand Names (USA)	Generic Name / Main Ingredient
Propulsid	Cisapride – No longer on the market in the USA. Limited availability in special circumstances
Bethanechol	Urecholine
Reglan	Metoclopramide
Motilium	Domperidone – Not available in the USA
Milk of Magnesia	Magnesium
Many brands	Erythromycin
Baclofen	Lioresal

Important information

All motility medications have a history of side effects and there are currently no great options for infants and children. Doctors are using them with a great deal of caution and looking forward to the newer motility medications that are currently being developed by several manufacturers.

Metoclopramide (Reglan) is in a class of medications called neuroleptics, which are used for control of vomiting, improvement of delayed gastric emptying and to treat serious mental illness such as schizophrenia. Metoclopramide has fallen out of favor due to the side effects and the mixed evidence about its effectiveness. Another use of metoclopramide is to increase milk supply in nursing mothers.

Bethanechol (Urecholine) is technically a medicine to help the bladder constrict and empty. Because it also works to constrict muscles in the digestive system, it can be used to improve motility. It does not come in a dose appropriate for children and must be compounded. The compound has a short shelf life. This drug is no longer commonly used in the US as a motility medication.

Cisapride (Propulsid) is no longer available in the USA. It was voluntarily pulled from the market by the manufacturer after patient deaths. It is still available for some patients under strict guidelines including EKG monitoring. It is being reformulated with the hope that it will be safer and more effective.

Baclofen (lioresal) is actually an anti-spasmodic that can be beneficial in reducing the number of inappropriate relaxations of the Lower Esophageal Sphincter. At present, this medication is most often used to treat children with muscle spasticity in addition to reflux disease. Some researchers are starting to try it for reflux alone.

Erythromycin is an antibiotic that causes diarrhea in typical doses. It can be used in small doses to improve GI motility. Taking antibiotics on a continuous basis is not the preferred way to treat reflux disease, but erythromycin is sometimes used if other options don't work. Researchers have been altering the molecular structure of this medicine to make it affect motility without also being an antibiotic. It will probably be available in the US as a motility medication in the next few years.

Milk of Magnesia is an antacid that causes diarrhea when taken in large doses. Small doses are sometimes used to improve GI motility.

Motilium (domperidone) is available in Canada and some US citizens import it for their children. Another use of domperidone is to increase milk supply in nursing mothers.

Side effects

Motility medications often cause mild side effect. They frequently cause abdominal cramps and diarrhea so the dose is often started low and increased slowly.

Metoclopramide side effects include: restlessness, fatigue, agitation, insomnia, headache, confusion, dizziness, depression, jitteriness, breast swelling, blood pressure changes, nausea, diarrhea, the need to urinate frequently and muscle spasms – particularly of the neck, voice box, tongue and eyes. Metoclopramide can cause serious neurological side effects, particularly in children. Parents need to discuss the side effects of this medication with the physician and pharmacist and weigh the benefit of using the medication vs. the potential for side effects. If your child is on this medication, ask for a list of the side effects so you can help watch for emerging problems. (I authored an article on these side effects that was published in Practical Gastroenterology and is available online from www.reflux.org.)

Bethanechol can cause bronchial constrictions and asthma attacks, a rapid heart rate, low blood pressure, whole body discomfort like the flu, abdominal cramps, nausea, belching, a sensation of overheating, constriction of the pupils and watery eyes.

Cisapride (Propulsid) was effective for some children, but it caused abnormal heart arrhythmias in some patients. After several deaths were reported, the manufacturer removed Cisapride from the market in the United States.

The current formulation of lioresal is sedating and may be habit forming, however, it is being reformulated.

Caution

This type of medication may change the rate of absorption of other medications so ask your doctor or pharmacist for assistance.

Anti-Gas Medications

Anti-gas medications reduce digestive gas production and disperse gas bubbles. While this class of medications is not truly a treatment for reflux, many babies experience painful burping and gas during and after a meal. Some doctors recommend this type of medication as part of a treatment plan for reflux.

Brand Names (USA)	Generic Name / Main Ingredient
Gas-X Mylanta Gas Mylicon Drops Phazyme	Simethicone

Practicalities

Simethicone seems to work well for some children but other parents report no relief.

Side Effects

There are no reported side effects.

Treatments for Related Symptoms

Medication to Increase Appetite

A medication to make your baby feel hungry or increase appetite is referred to as an appetite stimulant. This type of medication is not very common for treating reflux disease.

Brand Name	Generic name
Periactin	Cyproheptadine
Merinol	Marijuana derivative and not appropriate for children.
Megace	Similar to progesterone and not used in children.
Decadron	Dexamethasone is a synthetic steroid and not used in children.

Practicalities

Cyproheptadine (Periactin) is an antihistamine that has been used for increasing the appetite. The side effects may be significant and it is generally not used to treat reflux.

Side Effects

Cyproheptadine side effects include; dizziness, sleepiness, agitation, irritability, disturbed coordination, euphoria, hallucinations, fainting, rashes, low blood pressure, fast heart rate, dry mouth, anorexia, nausea, diarrhea, constipation, need to urinate frequently, difficulty urinating, wheezing, headache and chills.

Cautions

Periactin and H2 blockers both affect histamines and caution should be used when combining them.

Medication to Relax Muscles

Antispasmodic medications are used to relieve muscle cramps. This medication decreases the motion of the stomach and the intestines and the secretion of stomach fluids, including acid. The side effects may be significant and they are generally not used to treat reflux. This medication is commonly prescribed for "colic" in some parts of the US.

Brand Name (USA)	Generic Name
Donnatal	Belladonna with Phenobarbital

Side Effects

Donnatal is an anti-cholinergic medication that contains belladonna and Phenobarbital, a barbiturate used for epilepsy. The liquid elixir contains 23% alcohol. Side effects include sedation, dry mouth, inability to urinate, overheating, blurred vision, fast heart rate, loss of taste, headache, nervousness, insomnia, agitation, nausea, vomiting, constipation, body pain and rashes.

Medication to Reduce Nausea and Vomiting

An anti-emetic is a type of drug used to prevent and treat nausea and vomiting. The side effects may be significant and they are generally not used to treat reflux.

Brand Name	Generic Name
Compazine	Prochlorperazine – not for children due to significant neurological side effects and Reye Syndrome
Phenergan	Promethazine
Zofran	Ondansetron

Side Effects

Side effects of Promethazine include: sedation, neurological side effects such as tongue thrusting and eye rolling, elevated blood pressure, rash, nausea and vomiting.

Side effects of Ondansetron include: headache, diarrhea, constipation, dizziness, anxiety, agitation, slow heart rate, shivering, difficulty urinating, itching, low blood pressure.

Caution

Promethazine is an H1 histamine blocker and should be used cautiously in patients taking H2 histamine blockers.

Notes:

9 GIVING MEDICATION

Getting a prescription is just the first step to getting the medication into your child. This chapter has many ideas for getting your child to take the medicine without a fight. We also have ideas for proper measuring and other tips to help you be sure that the medicine works as well as possible.

Some medications need to be mixed and measured with a syringe; others need to be given with food or before a meal. It can be quite complicated to get started, especially if more than one medication is needed.

Different brands come in different formulations: tablet, capsule, time-release capsule, melt on the tongue tablet, powder and liquid. This variety should help you and your doctor find a formulation that you can get into your child successfully.

It is important to use each formulation the way the doctor and the pharmacist tell you to ensure that the medicine is absorbed effectively. The manufacturers have hotlines to answer questions about how to administer their medicines correctly.

Flavoring and compounding must also be done carefully according to strict recipes. Using the wrong flavoring can destroy the medication.

Do not increase the dose or stop giving the medication without consulting with the doctor. If your child is not responding to a medication, it is best to call the doctor or pharmacist for advice. Some medicines need to be withdrawn gradually rather than just stopped.

Use a special spoon or syringe to administer medications so your child does not associate her eating spoon with yucky tasting medicine. Try not to give medication in the high chair or use feeding utensils.

It is best to approach reluctant children in a straightforward, non-emotional tone, avoiding anger or punishments. Praise your baby when she cooperates. Offering rewards is often very effective.

Questions to ask the Pharmacist and Doctor

What type of medication is this (acid reducer, motility medication, etc)?

Will it take away all the symptoms or just improve them?

How long will it take to start seeing improvement?

When should I call or make a follow-up appointment to check on the success of treatment?

What is the exact dose of the medication?

Can I give medication without regard to food or meal times?

Are there special precautions with this medication in combination with other prescription or over-the-counter medications?

Are there any special instructions concerning how to use this medication?

Can it be flavored if my child hates it?

How long should I continue to give this medication?

What side effects should be reported?

How should I store this medication? Can I save unused portions for future use?

What should I do if I forget a dose of the medication?

Will the dosage need to be adjusted every time my child gains weight? How much weight? Do we need to come in or just call?

Always ask for the spelling of the drug and the dose and write it on the back of the prescription. Write down how many milligrams per kilogram so the pharmacist can check the math.

If we are supposed to use this medicine "as needed," how do we know when to use it?

If your child has a food allergy or intolerance, ask if there are any ingredients in this medicine that may cause problems.

Measuring Medication

Ask the pharmacist or nurse to show you how to measure the medication accurately. It is important to measure accurately. Even kitchen measuring spoons and most medication spoons are not accurate enough for pre-scription reflux medications.

You may need an oral syringe (with no needle) for your baby's medica-tion. To avoid squeezing the medicine out too fast, push the end of the plunger with the middle of your palm instead of pushing with your thumb or fingers. You have more control and can push slower.

> *I was using a thick syringe that the pharmacy gave me. It squirted the medicine into his mouth too fast and he would gag. Then he would cry and spit out a lot of his medicine, which meant that I never knew how much he was really getting. I asked the nurse at the hos-pital for a suggestion and she gave me a thinner syringe that pushes the medicine out slower. It worked perfectly!! Now he just drinks down the medicine without any fuss. And I must stress the words "without any fuss."*

There are several devices that can make it simpler to get the medicine out of the bottle and into your child. A MediBottle is a combination bot-tle and medication syringe that gives baby a squirt of medicine and a squirt of milk in the same mouthful. There are also special plugs called a press-in-bottle-adapter. It allows you to get liquid medicine into a sy-ringe without making a mess or spilling the bottle. Target offers these with all liquid medications. Other pharmacies may have them as well.

> *The pharmacist also gave me a special oral syringe top for the bot-tles so it makes it really easy to dose the medication.*

Adjust Dosage for Weight Gain

Some medications need to be adjusted for weight. The doctor will moni-tor growth and control of symptoms during follow-up visits and make dosing changes as needed.

> *It seemed like the medicine wasn't working any more. I asked the doctor to change to a medication that I heard about on the Internet. The doctor said we might eventually consider that medication, but for now, we should just try raising the dose a tiny bit. It worked! It turns out he had gained 2 lbs.*

◆

> *I write on the medicine bottle in BOLD print the current dose to be given...especially helps for those nights your eyes are not real wide-awake. Also, if grandma or a babysitter happens to come over to the*

*house they know exactly how much medication to give them. If we
have a dose increase, I cover the old dose with a large sticker and
write the new dose in large print.*

When it seems like your baby no longer needs medication for her reflux,
the doctor may slowly wean her off of the medication by keeping her
dose the same as she grows.

Pills and Capsules

Many reflux medicines only come in pills or capsules and a pharmacist
must make a form that an infant or child can take. A compounding
pharmacist can make them into a liquid "compound" with added sweet-
eners and anti-bittering flavorings.

Some medications come in a variety of forms including tablets, capsules, capsules with time-release beads of medicine inside, buffered tablets, micro-encapsulated (melt-in-your-mouth) tablets, microencapsu-
lated packets (powder to mix in water) and powder. Some even come in
IV forms.

Be sure to follow instructions from your doctor or pharmacist carefully
when giving the medicine to your child. If a medication comes in a pill
or capsule form, do not crush the pill or open the capsule unless given
specific instructions by the pharmacist. Do not cut tablets that are not
"scored" with an indented line. Crushing, splitting or opening pills and
capsules may ruin the effectiveness of the medication, especially a time
released medication such as a Proton Pump Inhibitor. Even packets of
powdered medicine and melt-in-your-mouth tablets are not designed to
be split into even doses.

Your pharmacist or doctor can call the manufacturer to learn how to
give these medicines without inactivating them. The instructions may be
different for each form and each brand.

A few medicines come in a dissolving form such as an efferdose tablet
that dissolves in your mouth. Some of these efferdose tablets can be
dissolved in water and the liquid can then be drawn into an oral syringe
and given to an infant.

*My four year old just started taking a new dissolving tablet. I told her
we were going try a new type of medicine that was magic. So we
made up a little routine: you put it on your mouth and then mommy*

will count to 10 and it will disappear on your tongue. She loves opening her mouth to say, "Ta Da!" when it is all gone. Of course, I made a huge deal about the magic for the first two weeks or so and made a point of saying to anyone that happened to be there (i.e. dad, grandparents)..."Watch we have a special magic trick that you won't believe." My daughter is very dramatic so I indulge that side of her by making a huge production out of things when I need her co-operation and it works really well for us!

Flavoring and Compounding

Does your child make a funny face or turn away when the medicine syringe is coming her way? It is possible that the medication has a terrible taste. Try a lick of the medication and see what you think. It is possible for the pharmacist to add special flavoring to the medication to mask even a strong flavor. Ask your doctor and pharmacist about custom mixing a compound that your child will take - no medicine works if you can't get it into the child.

Home flavorings such as chocolate syrup or jelly can reduce the effectiveness of some medicines, particularly PPIs.

I found a pharmacy that has tons of flavors. They were able to flavor one medication strawberry and the other grape. My daughter loved the flavors and took the medication so easily!

A compounding pharmacist can even make medication into lollipops or candy and give you a choice of two or three flavors. The consistency of the medication can be changed (thick to thin, thin to thick) and it can also be concentrated so you don't have to give such a large quantity.

There is a new flavoring system available to parents to flavor medicines at home. This is great for parents who can't find a local pharmacy that does the flavoring. It can also be used to flavor formula and over-the-counter medicines if needed.

Medications that have been compounded may lose their potency after a few weeks so ask your pharmacist for advice.

I noticed that my daughter's symptoms starting coming back when her compounded medication bottle was almost empty. When she had a fresh bottle of medication, her symptoms went away again.

*Finally, I realized that the medication was losing its strength and it
had to be made by the pharmacist more frequently.*

Not all flavorings can be used with all medications. Some flavors will
degrade some medicines and some flavors are not strong enough to
mask really nasty medicines. Ask your pharmacist before you promise
your child a certain flavor.

Your pharmacist can consult the International Association of Compounding Pharmacists for information on compounding and flavoring
medications. They have specific recipes.

*I highly recommend finding a compounding pharmacist. They have
gone so far as to make some of my son's meds taste like breast
milk when that's all he would take. The most recent success was to
get a nasty, thick antibiotic to taste like a thin fruit juice. He took it
right down.*

◆

*When we couldn't get our custom flavored medicine, the doctor
taught me to put my finger inside her mouth and hold her cheek
open while I used the syringe to put the meds toward the back of
her mouth. There aren't as many taste buds back there and she
could not spit the medicine out while my finger was in her cheek. He
also told me that sucking on an ice pop made of plain water can
numb her taste buds.*

While we want our children to have a good attitude about taking medicines, remember to be clear that they are not candy. Only adults should
give medicine and they need to be locked up at all times. Be careful
about keeping medicines in the diaper bag where a toddler can find
them. Toddlers will sometimes gobble the most disgusting medicines.

Timing

Some medications for reflux work more effectively if they are taken on
a precise schedule. Work with your doctor and pharmacist to make a
daily medication schedule.

Get advice when mixing medications with formula, foods or drinks
since this may alter effectiveness. For instance, grapefruit juice should
never be taken with any medication. Some medicines can't be mixed
with each other and should be given at different times of day.

Some medications work best if they are given 30 minutes before a meal so they have a chance to absorb. If you give them with food, they won't work as well.

Some children are more cooperative early in the day and less cooperative as they get tired. Ask your doctor about adjusting the timing of her dose if you think this could help.

Remembering to Give the Medicines

It is often difficult to remember to give the medication so parents often find creative ways to develop a routine.

If you want to use a high-tech solution, there are watches and beepers on the market that will sound an alarm at medication time. Your cell phone or PDA may have a function that can help you.

> *First, I would fill all of the syringes for the day. Then, I made a little line of syringes on the counter: two for the am, two at lunch, one at dinner and two at bedtime. It really gets easier when you develop your own routine. I kept the syringes in a shot glass and put it on a very high shelf.*

> *I have a wipe-off board that you can put on your refrigerator and a fancy kitchen timer/watch with four separate alarms. I keep a list of the doses and then check off as the day goes along. I found it to be a major brain saver!! Anything to help in those sleep deprived days!!!*

Common Questions and Concerns

Does My Child Need Medication?

Often, home care is enough to relieve the symptoms of reflux so it might be a good idea to try the basic treatments first. If the symptoms persist or cause worrisome side effects such as breathing problems or lack of weight gain, you and the doctor may decide to try a trial of medication.

Can I Use an Over-the-Counter Medication?

The antacid aisle of the pharmacy is brimming with over-the-counter medications for heartburn, stomach pain and other related conditions. It may be tempting to try a medication. After all, you don't need a prescription so how harmful can the medication be? The truth is, selecting a medication and determining the dose is best left to an experienced physician. Even over-the-counter medicines can be dangerous to some people in some circumstances. Any treatment begins with determining the diagnosis.

Your doctor will select a treatment such as a medication, taking into consideration both over-the-counter and prescription medications. Some medications are made for occasional use only and not for daily use for weeks or months. If you have seen a product on the pharmacy shelf or heard other parents discussing it, do not hesitate to ask the doctor or pharmacist if the medication is appropriate for your child.

What if I Don't Want to Give My Child Medication?

Some parents are uncomfortable with the idea of giving an infant or young child medication and prefer home treatment or a "natural" remedy.

I have to hold him upright all day and night. The doctor gave me a prescription for medication "just in case." For now, I would rather hold him day and night than give him the medication.

Many people believe that "natural" medicines such as herbs would be safer than prescription medications. Actually, most herbs have never been safety tested. (See the Chapter on Complementary and Alternative Medicine for info about herbs that are used for reflux.)

I asked my doctor about herbal of natural medicines. He asked me not to use them without his knowledge and consent. I was surprised to learn that some herbs are quite dangerous for babies. I guess I tend to think "natural" means "safe."

Be sure to discuss your concerns about medication with your doctor and ask for assistance in finding alternate remedies.

I only eat organic food and live a healthy lifestyle. There was no way that I was going to give my child medication at 6 weeks of age. By the time she was 10 weeks, we could tell that the esophagitis was worse than the side effects of the medication. We all agreed it was time to try medication.

What is the Strongest Medication Available?

After too many days spent comforting a crying baby, it may be tempting to think that a good, strong medication in a high dose will "fix" the reflux. If only it was that easy! While there are many good medications available, there is no treatment that is considered the best or strongest for every infant or child.

Generally, doctors choose the mildest medication that is likely to bring relief. They will "step up" to stronger medicines when needed, but will usually start with a low dose of a milder medication.

> *I'm sick and tired of this acid reflux. Just tell me the strongest medication available so I can tell my doctor to give me a prescription.*

If your baby has severe symptoms or has been suffering for a long time without treatment, the doctor may choose to use a strong medicine or a high dose to get her reflux under control quickly. After she has time to heal, the doctor may recommend that she "step down" to a lower dose or a milder medicine.

What Should I Do if My Baby Vomits Her Medication?

Ask the pharmacist or doctor if you should wait until the next dose or give the dose again. It is common for a baby to spit up or vomit when a new medication is introduced. However, if this happens each time you give the medication, the problem should be reported to the doctor right away. Your baby could be reacting to an ingredient in the medication such as a sweetener or a coloring. Or she might need to have a lower dose or a different medication.

Why Hasn't the Vomiting Stopped?

Most reflux medicines are designed to reduce acid, not stop the vomiting. Motility medicines can reduce the vomiting but they are not commonly used. Ask the doctor or the pharmacist to explain the type of medication your child is on and what to expect as a result of taking the medication. The goal is generally to stop all symptoms except the spitting up. Spitting up alone isn't usually a big concern as long as what comes up isn't acidic enough to burn and she isn't choking.

How do I know If My Child Still Needs the Medication?

It is important to have frequent office visits or phone consultations to evaluate the treatment plan. If your child seems to be feeling better, the doctor may gradually decrease the medication or stop increasing the dose. Sometimes, the doctor will ask you to stop the medication for one to two weeks to see if reflux symptoms return.

If your child had esophagitis or was refusing food, the doctor may want her to keep taking the medicine for several months to be absolutely sure she has time to heal.

Can it Help To Switch Brands?

A doctor may switch a child from one brand of medication to another if the child is not responding to the treatment. A hidden ingredient or difference in metabolism or some other reason may make your baby respond better to one brand.

> *The doctor told me that he likes brand A because it works better for most kids. Of course, brand B worked much better for my little one because she never follows any expectations.*

Not all insurance companies cover all brands of medications. Your doctor or the nurse may have to call the insurance company and get authorization to use a different brand. They may need to tell the insurance company that you tried the cheaper medicine and it didn't work.

Can I Mix the Medicine With Her Food?

Use caution when mixing medication into food or formula. The medication may not work as effectively when it is mixed with certain foods. In addition, an infant may dislike the new flavors or get full before finishing the food, thus reducing the overall dose given.

Is the Medication Safe?

The Food and Drug Administration approves a drug for use after the manufacturer submits data to prove that it is effective and safe in adults. They generally test the medication in about 500 adults.

When the FDA agrees that a drug is safe and effective it is then said to be "indicated" or "approved" for adults. It can still be used for children, but it has not been specifically tested in children.

Most of the reflux medicines on the market at the moment are tested in teens and approved for teens. Several of the reflux medications have been approved for infants and toddlers. Medication manufacturers are increasingly testing their medications and establishing safety and dosing recommendations for infants and children. This is vitally important because infants and children metabolize medication differently than adults and guessing the dose is not the best plan.

Often, reports of side effects come to the attention of the FDA after a medicine is already on the market. It is safest to use medicines that have been on the market several years because we know more about the safety. It is also wisest to choose medicines that have been used in children for several years. The best would be to use medicines that have been fully tested in children.

You and your doctor need to decide if the possible side effects of the reflux are more serious than the possible risks of taking the medication.

How Do I Report Problems with Medications?

If your child has had a significant problem with a medication, you should first discuss the situation with your child's doctor. Ask the doctor if the reaction was typical or unusual. Maybe the dose was miscalculated or the pharmacy gave you the wrong medicine.

You or the doctor may want to report medication problem to the Food and Drug Administration. Doctors are not required to report problems with medications, so you should feel free to do it yourself. The FDA states that over 90% of serious reactions are not reported. Reporting problems can prevent other babies from the same suffering.

Consumers may report problems to the Food and Drug Administration by phone at 1-888-463-6332, 800-INFO-FDA or on the web at www.fda.gov/medwatch. There is an on-line form or download the form and mail it to the FDA. You don't need to send medical reports or medical details. You don't need to 100% sure that what you saw was a side effect of a medicine. Just describe what you saw.

Notes:

10 Working with the Medical Team

It may seem really confusing to land in the world of medical care. You just became a parent. It feels like landing in a foreign country without a translator or guidebook. Even though you didn't sign up, you are about to go on the deluxe tour of the world of medicine with your sick baby. It will help if you take a crash course and learn a few tricks the experienced "travelers" have used.

This chapter will address many aspects of working with the medical team. There is a section on the specialists you might meet along the way and what they do. Most importantly, there are plenty of ideas on how to make the most of your medical appointments and keep all the team members working together smoothly.

Know Your Style

How you approach medical care with your baby is affected by the culture you grew up in, your past experiences with medical care, the way you view illness and how confident you are. You are going to be a very important part of the medical team. If you want to be the best team member you can be, it helps to understand how these influence the way that you work with the team.

Some people are raised in families where everyone is supposed to obey elders and authority figures without question. Other people are raised in families where questioning and heated debate of every topic is normal. Most families have a style in the middle of these extremes.

> *My husband gets upset when I ask questions because he thinks it looks like we don't trust the doctor. He wants to let the doctor make all of the decisions, but I want to be involved in the process. It must*

have something to do with authority figures because his family has arguments all the time about stupid things like the wind chill factor. And they certainly aren't shy.

The experiences of your family and friends during medical problems can greatly influence the way you work with the medical team. Any brushes with a missed diagnosis may have left you distrustful or even hostile toward doctors. Even long after you forgot all the details, the emotions may linger deep inside. A childhood memory of being held down by nurses may bring up fears that your child and the doctors can sense. Those fears can cause you to react emotionally instead of rationally.

Your childhood memories might focus on not fitting in with your peers when you were growing up. This can bring up fears of being different and make it tempting to avoid any medical diagnosis or treatment that could make your child feel different from other kids her age.

On the other hand, you may have great experiences with the medical world. You may have great confidence in the medical team and expect your doctor to know exactly what is wrong and how to fix it quickly. It is great to trust the medical team, but you might be disappointed that diagnosing reflux is not a perfect process and finding a treatment that works can involve some trial and error.

The way you view illness can also influence how you approach your baby's reflux. Do you feel that occasional, minor medical problems are just part of life or do you feel that each one needs to be solved right away? Neither attitude is right or wrong – it just helps to know where you fall on the spectrum.

The way you approach problems in general can also influence how you deal with your child's reflux. If you are a confident, take-charge person, you may feel very comfortable participating in medical decisions about your child's care and come into an appointment with an agenda and set of expectations. You may discuss the pros and cons of various treat-ments with the doctor, especially if you have already received your medical education from reading books or the internet! It may feel natu-ral to talk with the doctor and then make a decision.

I'm a very goal oriented person and so is my son's doctor. I love it when we lay out a plan of action together. This what we decided: 1. Start with a low dose of medication A. 2. Raise the dose a bit if needed. 3. When it seems to be right, bring him for a weigh-in every month and adjust medication. 4. If medication A doesn't work, we'll go to medication B. 5. If that doesn't work, we need to think about testing.

Some parents are shy about being part of the medical team. Remember, the doctor is depending on you to be his eyes and ears at home. Treating reflux is not an exact science. If you think the treatment isn't working, you need to report this so the doctor can try something new. Being shy isn't helpful when you have to talk for your baby. She can't tell the doctor what is going on – you have to.

Becoming an Educated Medical Consumer

It is important to make sure that you have a pretty good understanding of reflux. If you don't know much about reflux, you might not notice something about your baby that the doctor needs to know. Understanding the condition means understanding what each medication does or why you are keeping your baby upright after meals. It is not uncommon for parents to become very knowledgeable about pediatric reflux disease from signs and symptoms to medical treatments.

Most people do a better job of these tasks when they understand why they are important. All of your baby's family and caregivers should have a basic understanding of reflux so that they can help keep her as healthy as possible.

The internet offers a vast array of information and support websites to guide parents in their knowledge. Judging by the millions of visitors to the PAGER website at www.reflux.org, it is clear that parents are networking and searching for medical information.

My doctor likes it when I bring new articles and ideas to my appointment. He says I am his librarian!

Medical Jargon

Medicine is full of fancy words that are difficult to pronounce and doctors in different parts of the country use slightly different words or slightly different pronunciation. To make things more confusing, medical terms change over the years just like popular jargon

The long words or phrases get shortened. For example, a big label such as Gastroesophageal Reflux becomes GER, which some people say as separate letters and some people pronounce to rhyme with "her." When you read medical literature, you may run across the variation GOR. This is because the Brits spell it oesophagus but they pronounce it the same way we do.

At first, you may need to ask your doctor to slow down and speak in plain English. Soon, you will be speaking medical-ese yourself.

> *After a few months, I was an expert at all the jargon. I could tell the PCP (Primary Care Physician) that the Pedi GI (Pediatric Gastroenterologist) said the PPI (Proton Pump Inhibitor medication) needs to be increased 1 cc BID (twice a day) because the baby has increase her weight by a kilo (2.2 pounds). And add an H2 (acid reducer) PRN (as needed).*

If you are going to be reading medical journal articles, a good medical dictionary will be very helpful. You can also look up most words on the internet and find a definition. Beware that some words do not mean what people think they do. It is frightening to read about *morbidity* in an article until you realize it means illness, not death. Most people get the word confused with *mortality*, which does mean death.

Finding the Right Doctor

Most infants and children with reflux disease are treated by their primary care physician such as a family practitioner or pediatrician. These doctors are often called Primary Care Providers (PCPs) because they are the first person you go to for every problem and provide most of your care.

In some parts of the US and in many other countries, there aren't enough pediatricians to care for all the children in the area. In these places, pediatricians are considered specialists and only see children with complex medical conditions or developmental issues. Family practice doctors or nurses with advanced training are the Primary Care Providers for children who are basically healthy.

You and your child are going to be spending more time with the doctor than the typical pediatric patient. There may be extra phone consultations, office visits and weight checks. It is important to feel comfortable with the primary care physician and the office staff. You should feel that they take their time explaining things in a way that you can understand and they should really listen to you carefully.

> *The biggest lesson I learned in all this is to find a physician who trusts your intuition as a mother and will listen to it. I know it can be hard for doctors to always put all the pieces together, but we know our kids best and we need them to listen when things aren't right.*

The primary care office should have a telephone advice/call back system that is reliable so that you can relay information to the medical staff and receive a call back promptly, usually the same day that you call. You may want to talk with your doctor about the best time to call and how to handle an emergency after office hours. Do not hesitate to call during regular office hours for any problem, large or small.

The office staff and nurses should be respectful and courteous to you, even if you are a frequent customer. Caring for a child with reflux can change from day to day and it is common to have frequent questions and concerns.

> *When we were searching for a pediatrician, I paid as much attention to the staff as I did to the doctors. One unhappy nurse or office manager can ruin a visit or can blow off a small problem until it becomes an emergency. Efficient, friendly staff who know the kids names and have been with the practice for years can make your visits a lot smoother.*

Ideally, the primary care physician will be the main doctor helping to coordinate care, especially if other specialists are involved. Be sure to ask the specialists and others (radiology, blood lab, etc) to forward test results to the primary doctor. That way, your main doctor will have all of the information needed in one place to make the best medical decisions.

If your child has very complex reflux complications, the pediatric gastroenterologist may want to help with case management. Ask the pediatric GI if he wants to see the reports from any other specialists and help coordinate care.

Who Are All of These Specialists?

Your primary care physician may suggest that your child see a specialist if she has complications of reflux or doesn't respond to treatment. If possible, select a specialist with pediatric training. A children's hospital or clinic may be a good place to find a specialist.

> *After a long wait, we finally got to see the Pediatric Gastroenterologist for the first time. What a relief. When I gave him the medical history he kept nodding in understanding that all of it was related to reflux. I cannot begin to tell you how relieved it made me.*

Pediatrician: Doctor specializing in the care of children from newborns to adolescents.

Pediatric Gastroenterologist: A doctor who is trained first as a pediatrician and then receives additional training in children's diseases of the gastrointestinal tract.

Pediatric Pulmonologist: A medical doctor with additional training in lung diseases affecting children such as asthma and sleep apnea.

Pediatric Otolaryngologist or Ear, Nose and Throat Doctor (ENT): A doctor with training in diseases of the ears, nose and throat such as ear infections, sinus infections, voice problems and upper airway issues.

Pediatric Allergist: A medical doctor with specialized training in pediatric allergic diseases such as food and environmental allergies.

Dietician / Nutritionist: A nutritionist addresses diet and nutrients (vitamins and minerals) needed to ensure health and growth. They know how age, illness and lifestyle affect nutrition and provide counseling and encouragement. Not all medical school programs teach nutrition thoroughly.

Speech Language Pathologist: This professional can diagnose and treat problems with swallowing, oral motor issues, language comprehension and speech.

Occupational Therapist: This professional can help with sensory processing, developmental skills, feeding issues, and provide parent education.

Physical Therapist: This professional can help children who have low muscle tone or high muscle tone which can aggravate reflux. Many will also work with children who have developed poor posture because their stomach pain causes them to slouch.

Neonatologist: A pediatrician specializing in the treatment of newborns and premature babies. Many also treat former preemies as they grow.

Developmental Pediatrician: A doctor who specializes in children with neurological and developmental problems and complex medical issues. Many have certifications in developmental and behavioral pediatrics.

Hospitalist or Intensivist: This person is a doctor who works full time at a hospital and is responsible for the care of children who are staying overnight. This doctor coordinates with the primary care physician. A hospitalist who cares for children will probably be trained as a pediatrician with extra training in intensive care.

Lactation Consultant: Lactation consultants teach breastfeeding and can help both babies and moms learn the skills to make this successful.

Medical Social Worker: Medical social workers provide counseling for families who are dealing with a significant illness and help them find the practical resources they need. They may work for local government agencies, hospitals or home health agencies.

Counselor, Psychologist, Psychiatrist: All of these professionals can provide advice and counseling. Psychiatrists can prescribe medications to treat depression and other mood problems and have more training in diagnosing and treating mental illness.

Pediatric Dentist: A specialist with several additional years of training after dental school. The pediatric dentist is concerned with the overall health of the child. They treat infants to teens and often continue to treat patients with special needs after they are adults. They take great care to alleviate pain and fear in their patients and the parents.

Pediatric Nurse Practitioner: This nurse has advanced training beyond the basic nursing training and most states allow the PNP to provide all basic care including medication as long as they work closely with a doctor.

Physician Assistant: This professional receives training to do most of the same things a pediatrician does. In some states, they are allowed to prescribe medications. A PA is supervised by a doctor.

Feeding Team: An infant or child with a feeding disorder may be referred to a feeding team. A clinic or hospital may have a group of doctors and specialists such as a Pediatric Gastroenterologist, a lactation consultant, speech therapist, occupational therapist, nutritionist and psychologist who work together to diagnose and treat feeding problems and related behavioral issues.

Practical Tips for Appointments

Spending a few minutes getting organized before a doctor's appointment, can help you get the most out of the appointment and make it go smoother. It is always a terrible feeling to leave an appointment and think, "Oh no! I forgot to tell the doctor something!"

Before the appointment:

Line up your referrals from your primary care doctor at least a week ahead of time. Preferably, two weeks.

Make a list of symptoms you are seeing at home. Place a star next to the top 3 worrisome symptoms. These are the symptoms you really want to address with the doctor.

Prepare a journal with a 3-day record of symptoms, food intake, sleep patterns, etc.

Make a list of the medications

Several days before the appointment, start making a list of questions so you will not forget to ask something important. Ask your spouse and friends to help you remember things you said you wanted to ask the doctor next time.

Talk to an experienced parent and get help clarify your list of questions and go over the journal to look for patterns.

During the appointment:

Tell the doctor you have a list of questions and make sure you have the opportunity to go through your entire list. If the doctor is getting ready to end the appointment, you can remind him/her that you have a few more questions.

Record your answers. When you leave the appointment, you should know the diagnosis, the next treatment, a plan for follow up with the doctor or staff and how to reach the doctor with questions and concerns.

I always have a pad of paper and pen, to write down anything the doctor says that I need to remember. That way he knows I am serious. I also repeat certain things that she says: "So, you are saying this..."

It may be helpful to bring another adult with you such as a relative or friend. This person can help you ask questions, make suggestions, write down information and help juggle the baby so you can talk.

Record Keeping

Doctors like hard data. At each appointment, your doctor will most likely ask you specific questions such as, "How many ounces of formula were consumed each day?" How many times did she vomit?" etc. If you are already exhausted from limited sleep, it may be difficult to remember what happened an hour ago, much less last week.

Dear PAGER Parent Volunteer, We saw the pediatric gastroenterologist on Monday and did get a diagnosis of gastroesophageal reflux. I followed your advice and very carefully charted his day for three days, which greatly helped. I also spent hours preparing a one-page sheet of my top three concerns and all the symptoms that went with the concerns. If I hadn't contacted you, I am fairly certain I would have collapsed into a frustrated crying heap in his office; but instead, I was calm because I felt prepared. As a result, the doctor has doubled the amount of medicine that my baby takes and we will start another medicine in three weeks if needed. I feel so much better now that we have a plan!

Use a system that allows you to write down information quickly. For instance, if you have to give a medication three times a day, write down the name of the medication and place a check next to it after you have given each dose. This will help you remember to give the meds as well as give you a record to bring to the doctor.

Many parents like a hardbound diary or spiral notebook to write down information. Some parents create a blank chart or spread sheet and print a copy every day. During the day, they record notes on it. At the end of the day, you can put the chart in a three ring binder or slip it into a folder that closes. Use something that will hold the papers securely if you drop it.

We have provided sample charts in the back of this book. They may not work for you. If you create a different chart, please send a copy to Beth@refluxbook.com so we can share it with other parents.

Use your notebook or chart to write down the details that are important to your child's care - medication, vomiting episodes, how much food you offered and how she ate, how much came back up, wet diapers, messy diapers, amount of crying and now much she sleeps.

> Writing everything down has helped me. I found that when I wrote down how often my daughter rejected food or a bottle it really appeared quite alarming. I write down every incident of discomfort she seems to have.

It is always a good idea to get copies of test results and summary letters that the doctors send each other. Many doctors and labs now automatically send a copy of these to the patient or their parents.

There are many companies that help you create a secure, personal medical record to keep all the important information online. You can give full or limited access to each doctor you see.

If the reflux persists over time, you may find yourself describing the problem to a variety of doctors and specialists. You may want to take a moment to write a one-page summary with the following information: diagnosis, tests, illnesses, current medications and doses, plus a growth chart.

> My handwriting was so messy that there was no way the doctor would be able to make sense of the notebook I had been keeping in the diaper bag – besides, it smelled like vomit. I spent an hour copying the information more clearly. Not only was it easier to read, it helped me to look at the entries more closely and see patterns I wasn't able to see in the mess. Sometimes, I would have another person look at it and they would be able to spot patterns that I just couldn't see. My friend noticed that my baby seemed to spit up a lot more on days when she didn't have a BM.

As the reflux gets better, you may find that keeping daily records is too much work. Once in a while, pick a day and record symptoms and feedings, etc. Pick a day when you think you will be sticking to your typical schedule. If your child has an unusual day, start over the next day. Comparing one "typical" day each month can help you observe patterns and see progress.

> *About once a month, I would write down all of the foods my toddler ate in a day. I could compare her eating from a month or even 6 months ago and see such big changes. Perhaps she had increased the amount of food she ate at one meal or started eating food from another food group. In the day–to-day struggles, it was hard to see that we were making progress in her eating but the record showed she was eating and drinking more over time.*

Common Frustrations with the Medical System

You may be finding out the hard way how the medical system works. You may need pre-authorization for tests and treatment as well as co-pays and rules to follow. Some insurance companies require that a primary doctor such as a pediatrician serve as the gatekeeper for medical care.

Medical care has changed and continues to change at a rapid rate. The reality is, you may not see the same practitioner all of the time if you are part of a big practice. Doctors face limitations from insurance companies and complex rules for authorization of treatment and even which medications to prescribe. Many doctors do not have as much time as they want to see patients.

> *My baby goes to a group of five pediatric gastroenterologists in a big city. The logistical stuff they have to deal with is so overwhelming that they hired one nurse just to do medication refills and deal with the insurance companies. A friend in another part of the country says her GI office has a reflux nurse who only deals with the reflux families.*

> *I couldn't believe that I had to wait so long to get an appointment with the Pediatric Gastroenterologist. I called another hospital an hour away and the wait was even longer.*

Sometimes you will get lucky and find a pediatrician who still manages to spend lots of time with patients who are having a rough time. This is wonderful but don't be disappointed if it doesn't happen.

> NO ONE understood what we were going through except our doctors - thank God we had a great pediatrician who had just come back from maternity leave and had a reflux baby of her own. She called us every day – I think she was checking on us more than the baby!

Coordinating care between multiple doctors can be another source of tension. Doctors don't get paid for the time they spend coordinating care and this can be very time consuming if your baby has lots of visits to specialist or therapists.

Insurance companies and managed care organizations are limiting the amount of time that the doctor can spend with each patient. Your doctor may have patients scheduled every ten minutes and seem rushed or respond slowly to your phone message.

In many offices, you don't always see the same doctor at every visit. You may get tired of explaining things to a new doctor, but once in a while, the other doctor may notice something somebody else missed. You can view this as a problem or as a chance to get a second opinion without much hassle. Sometimes doctors who work together have very different styles and training.

> My doctor reviewed my daughter's chart with another doctor in the practice because she has a complex case. If my primary doctor is out of the office, I can usually schedule with the other doctor. It saves me from explaining the whole complex history to an unfamiliar member of the practice and ensures we get more coordinated care.

At times, it may feel like you are the case manager. It may be assumed that you know all of the lab results and weight/height measurements so the doctors may look to you for this information. While it may seem like the doctors should have all of the information at their finger tips, the reality is that you may be the one with the most information. Don't hesitate to speak up and give information that may guide the doctor. All of the little clues can add up and help the doctor make the best decision.

When You and the Doctor are Not on the Same Page

Often, when a parent is frustrated with the doctor, it is a problem of communication. When a parent talks to a PAGER Association parent volunteer, the volunteer may ask questions to clarify a parent's concerns and help to identify the main concern or issue. If the parent expresses multiple concerns, the parent volunteer will ask a parent, what is your biggest worry or concern? By clarifying the problem and listing questions, the parent is ready to talk with the doctor.

Before appointments, I prepare a list of my questions and fax it to the doctor. It makes me get organized and gives the doctor time to review the chart to see if tests are back, etc. Then the doctor can keep the fax in the chart.

This is a story about two babies with the same symptoms. Each parent brings the baby to the doctor. However, each parent communicates with the doctor in a very different way. See what happens.

Parent A says, "My baby cries and spits up all the time." The doctor thinks, "I hear this from every parent of a new baby." The doctor tells the mother, "Watch him and let me know if it gets worse. It is common for babies to cry and spit up in the newborn period."

Parent B opens her book and starts reading. "During the last three days, my baby cried 12-16 hours a day, vomited 1-2 ounces at each feeding and she wants to nurse 10-12 times a day." The doctor thinks, "I need to ask this parent more questions and find out why this baby is in such terrible pain."

Which baby gets better care? It is likely that the first parent will go home thinking, "That doctors doesn't get it," while Baby B will get a thorough exam following an in-depth discussion between the parent and the doctor. In addition, the second parent is likely to go home with a treatment plan and instructions for follow up. Both the baby and the parents will be happier.

My pediatrician was a very mellow guy. I usually appreciate this, but I felt he wasn't paying enough attention to my son's poor weight gain. I asked him to write in the chart that "mom is very concerned about baby's weight and I blew her off." That got his attention. We went over my son's weight chart and it was worse than the doctor realized. It turns out he was mistaken about my son's age.

Second Opinions – Getting a Fresh Perspective

Sometimes it is necessary to bring your child to another doctor. A second opinion provides an opportunity to get a fresh perspective on the situation or develop a new treatment plan.

Perhaps you need a practitioner with different training or a personality style that meshes better with your family's needs. Maybe you like the doctor you see now, but this time you are looking for a doctor who is willing to experiment with the newest treatment options because you have already tried all the standard treatments and they didn't work well enough for your baby.

Getting a second opinion is recommended before a major change in treatment such as surgery, a feeding clinic or tube feeding. Some insurance companies even urge patients to get second opinions before surgery.

Reflux is common enough that you should be able to get an independent opinion without traveling too far. If your child has a rare or unusual problem related to reflux, it may be necessary to see a specialist in another part of the country.

Did you know that a doctor's favorite treatment often depends on who his teachers were? If your doctor's internships and residency were at a medical facility where Drug A was often used, he is likely to try that one first because that is what he is most comfortable with. If you get a second opinion from a doctor who trained in a different place, you might learn that Drug B or even surgery are higher on his list.

Being a Good Patient

If you are having some problems working well with the doctor or staff, be sure that you are doing what you need to do to make things work smoothly.

It helps the office staff and doctor if a single family member is the designated contact person. Calls from more than one parent can overburden the staff and create miscommunication.

Part of being a good patient is keeping your appointments and being on time. Even if you are kept waiting every time, you still need to arrive on time for the appointment.

It is very difficult for doctors to work with parents or patients who make medical decisions and inform the doctor later. Deciding not to take the medicine, changing the dose or other making changes in what the doctor prescribed should only be done after talking to the doctor.

If you are lucky, your child's doctor may take on a support role to you and your family. Remember, it is the PRIMARY job of the doctor to provide medical care for your child.

While it is important to be informed, remember to be a good listener and hear what the doctor has to say. Your doctor has experience treating other patients with similar problems and has a good idea of how to proceed.

When I talk with pediatricians, they complain that many parents of their patients are demanding medication, even for minor reflux. Yet when I talk with parents, they complain that the doctors don't provide a treatment plan that addresses the significant symptoms they see at home.

Be sure to call the doctor if the treatment isn't working. The doctor will assume that all is well unless you call to say it isn't.

Wanting to Change Doctors?

You may reach a point where you feel it is time to switch doctors. There may have been a single incident that triggers the need to move on. Or perhaps there were a series of events over time such as on-going communication issues.

> It wasn't until I switched doctors that I realized what an outstanding doctor looked like. I was so impressed when the new doctor spent about an hour going over my daughter's complex history. I could tell he was really listening and took my concerns very seriously. He is an excellent problem solver and really gets to the root of the problem. I know that I can count on him and I really value his judgment.

Unfortunately, you may not have an abundant choice of doctors if you live in a rural area. Even in large cities, there are not enough pediatric gastroenterologists. You have the challenge of either resolving your differences to make the situation better, or traveling a long distance to another city or out of state for care.

You may be forced to stay with your current doctor if you have insurance coverage that limits your options or other logistic reasons. There are several ideas that might help you improve the working relationship with your doctor.

It may help to make an appointment just to talk about the communication issues between you. Leave the baby home if you can. Ask if you can schedule a longer appointment if your child has complex needs.

Your primary care physician may be able to help sort thing out or run interference. You can also ask for help from a medical ombudsman who is trained to help medical consumers work out problems. Hospitals generally have an ombudsman and the state insurance commissioner probably has one. Your insurance company might have an ombudsman. Your local hospital may have a family services coordinator or you may be able to get assistance from the child life department or the hospital chaplain. You can also hire a private patient advocate. Many are nurses.

Consider having your spouse or a carefully chosen friend come with you to an appointment. It is best to find somebody calm, logical but very firm. Look for somebody who likes to make things better, not somebody who will add to the problems.

> *I didn't feel that the appointments with the doctor were very productive. I was so sleep deprived that I wasn't thinking clearly. I'm sure my appearance didn't help me be taken seriously – the barf on my wrinkly clothes just didn't command respect. We got a lot more attention and time the day my husband came with me in his suit and carrying his briefcase filled with spreadsheets documenting the number of baby barf episodes.*

Go back to the doctor and get answers your questions. If the doctor makes you feel like a silly worrier, just say to your self, "my baby needs me to know as much as I can to help her. I am in the front line and must trust my instincts." Tell that doctor that you don't feel like your concerns have been taken seriously.

> *Seek out a doctor who is sympathetic to your needs as a mother and who makes you feel secure in his care. And who LISTENS TO*

YOU. I firmly believe that a doctor who leaves you feeling confused or insecure is not doing a very good job. Mother and child are a unit and should be treated as such.

Remember, you know your child best and so you are in the best position to make decisions for her. You need to be respectful and courteous when talking to the doctor and office, but stand your ground when you feel that further treatment is needed. You are your baby's best advocate. Be persistent and diplomatic. Make them listen to you

I have found that educating myself and taking matters into my own hands has proven to be the most effective. I know what is working for her and what is not and that there really is a true maternal instinct with stuff like this.

◆

The notebook I was keeping didn't seem to be enough to convince the pediatrician that my daughter was having serious problems. I took a video of my daughter during an attack and I took the camera in for the pediatrician to watch. I don't think he appreciated it very much but it made my point and I was at Pediatric GI the next day. Surprise - she has severe reflux. Sometimes you just have to make a big statement.

If you find that the doctor is not providing the type of reassurance and support that you need as a parent, contacting a patient support organization such as PAGER Association can make a huge impact.

I was pretty angry and disillusioned at the medical system by the time I found PAGER Association. After I met some other parents who really understood what I was going through, I began to realize that I was expecting too much of the doctors. They were providing excellent care for my son. I stopped looking to the doctors for emotional support because I had a circle of reflux moms to listen and support me.

If you find it is best for your baby to change doctors, try not to burn your bridges. If your insurance changes or the new doctor leaves town, you may end up back where you started. It may be best to "fire" the doctor by writing a letter rather than risking a heated argument. Try to stick to the facts when you let the doctor know you are moving to another practice.

Notes:

11 INTENSIVE CARE PARENTING

At PAGER Association, we coined the term *Intensive Care Parenting* to describe the high level of parenting necessary to care for a child with reflux. Taking care of a *high need* baby 24/7 can leave you feeling stressed and exhausted most of the time. Babies with reflux can wear out even the most seasoned parent.

Think of this chapter as a virtual support group. You will hear the voices of other parents who share your fears and isolation. Often, it is a relief to find that others share our struggles.

If reading about the stress of reflux is too depressing, skip ahead to the Coping Tips section for some parent-tested ways to cope with the day-to-day parenting issues of reflux.

How Hard Is It?

Intensive Care Parenting is being on call 24/7. Feeding, comforting, mixing medication and formula, going to doctors appointments and cleaning spit-up. You also perform a hundred other little tasks too numerous to mention. The work is endless. Your back aches and you are constantly in a state of exhaustion. You can't remember the last time you slept in your bed, much less had a full night of sleep. You seldom get a break from your role.

We have received desperate calls on the PAGER warm line from physicians, PhD's and pediatricians who tell us that parenting their child with reflux has been the hardest thing they have done. One veteran New York City police officer/parent told us she would rather walk the beat than stay up all night with her screaming baby! Several pediatricians said they knew that babies with reflux are hard to care for but they didn't realize that it was this bad.

Your whole body may ache from holding and carrying your inconsolable baby. It is hard work to bend and lift, vacuum and load the washing machine with a baby on your shoulder or in a carrier. You may be in a state of exhaustion from a full day of caretaking only to face frequent night waking for more feeding, holding and comforting. The nights can feel very long.

Everyone tells you to "sleep when the baby sleeps" but this may not be practical if the baby doesn't sleep or sleeps on an erratic schedule. It is always tempting to try to run around and get things done during those fleeting moments when the baby is sleeping. It may be the only time the baby is not attached to you!

> *My 10-week-old baby didn't even take a nap during the day. Occasionally, she would pass out for 15-20 minutes after a really bad crying spell. She seldom slept more than 2 or 3 hours at night before waking up again. How was I supposed to "sleep when the baby sleeps" if she was wide-awake all day?*

Most of the night duty falls on the shoulders of mothers, especially breastfeeding moms. Even with the help of a supportive spouse, the long-term consequences of interrupted sleep can include mental confusion, depression and moodiness. You may also have a difficult time focusing and remembering things.

Negative Feelings

You may feel that the initial joy and euphoria from childbirth has been quickly replaced with a dark cloud of frustration, anxiety and exhaustion. This may unfold as the days and week's progress and your baby begins to experience more pain and discomfort.

We all read the baby books while we were pregnant, so we knew that sleep deprivation and care taking were part of the parenting package deal. We read that babies cry, spit-up, mess their diapers and do other unpleasant things. We also read that we would bond with our babies and love every minute of feeding and hugging.

So what happened? While the other moms were dressing their babies in Baby Gap matching outfits and meeting friends for lunch at the coffee shop, we ended up at home, in formula and spit-up stained clothes, holding a fussy baby with tears streaming down our cheeks. The other moms got tickets to the "Parenting by the Book Tour" while you get to ride on the "Reflux Rollercoaster."

You are not alone. Your feelings are very normal and expected under the circumstances. You will find other companions in your journey. Somewhere in the distant future, you may even be surprised to hear yourself say, "It was hard, but we survived it and it made us stronger."

My story: There is one benefit to having a child with reflux – you pay such close attention when she is little, that you end up knowing her better when she is older. It can take several months to catch on, but you end up knowing her moods as well as her health. I can tell when my daughter is getting sick several hours before she gets a fever because her voice changes. Nobody else can hear the difference, but I'm right every time. Even the pediatrician agrees to put off immunizations when I say I think Katie is getting sick. When Katie was little, I used to tell her, "When you are 27 years old and have purple hair and tattoos, you can still come home and sit on my lap whenever you want to." At seventeen, has a very independent personality, but she still wants me to lie in her bed and watch TV with her when she doesn't feel good. I don't think this closeness would have happened without reflux and all those months we spent practically joined at the hip.

Disappointment

You may feel disappointed that your plans to be a super mom with a perfect baby have been replaced by the grim realities of smelly vomit covered clothes on both you and the baby and deep lines of stress and fatigue on your face.

You may have feelings of disappointment when several months go by and she still has reflux. Sometimes the doctor will tell you, the baby will outgrow the reflux when he sits up or by one year of age. As parents, we mark our calendars, waiting for the reflux to go away!

When he turned 6 months of age, I was a little disappointed that he hadn't outgrown his reflux. I was sure he would outgrow it by one year of age. At his one-year-old birthday, he wouldn't even eat his cake because he is a picky eater and only tolerates pureed food. I felt sad and depressed. I felt so cheated. When would the reflux ever end? I felt depressed for weeks after his birthday.

◆

I had expected to take home my perfect baby boy and spend my days cuddling and enjoying him. I couldn't believe it when he cried almost non-stop. This isn't the way it is supposed to be I thought to myself. I felt bad for him, of course, but I also felt sorry for myself. I had wanted everything to be perfect, and what I actually had was a screaming, sick little boy. Part of me was sad I didn't get the child I thought I wanted. Then, I felt guilty for feeling that way.

Guilt

You may look back on the pregnancy and delivery for clues about what you did to "cause" the problem. Did I eat too much acidic food? Was it the medication at childbirth? Is there something wrong with my milk? As far as we know, you did not do anything to "cause" your baby to have reflux.

You may find yourself yearning for the old days before this baby was born – Before Reflux (B.R.). A tiny part of you wishes you could go back to your old life.

Don't get me wrong, we love our new baby so much, but it does make me long for the one-on-one time with our other daughter. I got pregnant when my older daughter was only 8 months old. I sometimes feel a little bad because all the happiness and joy we had with my older daughter is pretty much gone. Our time is spent in doctor's offices, hospitals and pacing the floor with a crying infant. I look at our happy toddler and feel tremendous guilt about what we can't give her in terms of our time. We used to laugh and play. Now we just try to get through the day with our sanity intact. My husband and I get short with each other a lot because we are just both so tired of being tired. The joy we so longed for in becoming parents was short-lived. Now each day is long and exhausting with very little fun.

It is hard to bond with a baby who is miserable. You were looking forward to a peaceful time snuggling with a baby who has that sweet baby smell.

It's almost impossible to bond with a reflux baby at first. Even our pediatrician said "who can bond with something that screams at you all day??"

Overwhelmed

When you entered the world of parenting, you knew that you would be busy taking care of your little bundle of baby and have to learn a whole new language of breastfeeding and umbilical cord care. You didn't expect that you would have to get a whole medical education, adding fancy terms to your vocabulary such as pediatric gastroenterologist and Gastroesophageal reflux. Just when you had mastered skills like changing diapers and holding a floppy newborn, you had to learn to measure medications, modify your diet and learn 27 ways to soothe a very unhappy little baby.

Taking care of a fussy baby can consume most of your time, making it difficult if not impossible to take care of your basic needs such as eating, sleeping and bathing. The house is a mess, the bills haven't been paid and you can't imagine how you will find the time to go to the grocery store.

I remember going for days without washing my hair - when the baby spit up in my hair, I just held that section under the kitchen faucet.

My daughter is extremely bonded with me, devastated when I leave for work, is often clingy and can make it extremely hard for me to accomplish anything around the house. I honestly think some of our wonderfully close (and sometimes draining) bond is due to the fact that she spent so much time in pain that I was one of her only sources of comfort for so long.

Anger and Frustration

You may feel anger toward those you love and need the most- your spouse, your family and your friends. You may even feel angry at your baby. You have no control over your life. Everything is too hard. No one understands.

One night she kept waking up every 30-45 minutes. I would nurse her and she would fall asleep on my chest. Every time I placed her back in her crib, she would instantly wake up and start crying again. This went on for about 3 hours. I felt my anger rising. I was losing control. I was so tired, I just couldn't function another minute. I woke up my husband and asked him to hold her. I didn't tell him, but at that moment, I felt like I could hurt her.

You may lash out at anyone in your path You find yourself angry and frustrated at everybody – your spouse, your mother-in-law, your sister-in-law with the perfect baby, the doctor, the nurses, the idiot driver in front of you, your toddler. Even your baby.

My story: My low point came the day that Katie spilled a bottle of custom compounded medication that was very expensive and hard to get. I walked out of the house and handed her to a complete stranger. All I knew about the woman was that she had kids and lived in the house on the corner. At that moment, I felt she could take better care of my baby than I could. I couldn't make my baby stop crying and I couldn't feed her right. My poor toddler, Chris, was a mess and acting up because he missed his mommy who was always busy with that shrieking baby. I felt like the worst mother in the world. I was worried if I had to drive back the pharmacy, I might drive into a tree - on purpose.

A Word about Shaken Baby Syndrome
Sometimes a baby can make you feel a level of anger you never thought was possible. Fatigue and frustration can build up and in a moment of rage, the baby may become the focus of your anger. Parents have been known to shake or smack a baby in an attempt to stop the crying. Shaking a baby can leave the child in a wheelchair, cause blindness, brain damage and even death.

If you feel that your anger is rising to a dangerous level, you need to take immediate action:

Put your baby in a safe place such as a baby seat or crib and go to another room. Turn on the shower or radio so you can't hear the crying.
Call someone to come over right away – spouse, friend or neighbor.
Seek medical care – perhaps your baby is crying due to an ear infection, thrush or some other illness.

Put the baby in a car seat and drive – perhaps the car ride will be soothing to your baby.

Call your local community hotline and find out if there is a "crisis nursery" in your area – a free, safe place to leave your child for up to 72 hours.

Go to a store, fire station or 24 hour restaurant. Find somebody who will take a turn holding and comforting your baby and let you sit in your car and cry – alone.

When my baby drives me to the brink, I put myself in time-out by locking myself in the bathroom. It is much healthier than directing my anger at her!

Misunderstood

Doesn't it seem like every time you complain to the doctor about how much your baby is crying she sleeps during the entire appointment? You just want to scream if one more person tells you, "She looks so healthy," "She will eat when she is hungry," "My child did the same thing," or "Why don't you just let her cry it out?"

No one seems to understand what it is like to take care of this little child with acid reflux. You get tired of explaining it and explaining why you are having such a hard time.

◆

Everybody asks, "Is she a good baby?" With my first, I was afraid to say, "NO." I didn't want them to know I was a horrible mother who didn't like her baby who vomited and screamed all the time. When my second child was born, I knew better. I could tell everyone with a laugh, "No. I have miserable babies, but they grow into great kids!"

Isolated

You may find that you barely leave the house because you are so tired and it is just too much work. You may also dread running into other moms who have perfect babies or seeing relatives and friends who don't understand. You may find that you even take the phone off the hook because the noise might wake the baby from her precious 20-minute nap.

My son sleeps very poorly during the day and screams a lot so I avoid taking him out. I went shopping with him one day - I could see all the people staring at me, certain they were thinking, "does that lady KNOW her baby is screaming?" while I browsed seemingly un-affected through the clothes rack). My bedtime is 8 pm so I can't even meet friends after both kids are in bed, and during the day, I'm just too busy with the baby. If I get out of the house without the baby, I have to take my toddler so my husband isn't home with both of them, so that's not much of a break, either!!!

You cannot face going to the moms club or sharing your story with other parents. They just don't seem to get it. None of them have an in-consolable baby who spits-up and arches. Your relatives tell you no other family member acted like this during infancy - all of the other grand babies ate and slept just fine. You feel like the only parents in the history of the universe to have such a difficult baby.

Most parents feel lucky when friends have babies the same age. We feel unlucky that several of our friends do. If their baby cried for 30 minutes, hey were worried about colic. Ha!- 30 min. compared to 15 hours a day!? It was SO SO hard to see others with their non-reflux babies.

Scared

Many parents experience a high level of fear when their baby is sick. If a normal parent drives at 80 miles per hour to the emergency room for a little cut, it is no wonder parents of a child with reflux get panicky sometimes.

Sometimes the fear is related to not knowing what comes next. Some parents find that learning more about the condition can make them feel less scared. Other parents find that reading about reflux just puts more scary possibilities into their minds. They are like medical students who suddenly start to think every headache could be brain cancer. The more they know about medicine, the more scared they get.

I knew I was being irrational but I just didn't care. My daughter's re-flux wasn't bad at all, but I somehow convinced myself that she was going to die. I knew I was being a hysterical mom, but the more they tried to shut me up, the more hysterical I became. Everybody told me that sleep would help me be calmer – they didn't know that my sleep was full of nightmares about losing the baby at the store (she can't walk yet) or kidnappers taking her and holding her for ransom (we don't have a spare dime).

You may also find that you go into a mode where your fear is so great that your brain just turns it off.

> *My baby choked and we called 911. A few seconds later, she started breathing again. While my husband comforted her, I started looking for a cute outfit to change her into so the EMT's would think I was a good mother. When my husband asked what I was doing, I realized how absurd it was. Stress and fear often make me do strange things.*

Embarrassed

Having a child who is sick all the time can make your feel embarrassed and different. You don't invite people over because house is a mess. You are worried about letting anybody hold the baby because she always throws up on the most expensive outfit in the crowd. Maybe you used to be well dressed at all times and even wore matching clothes to the grocery store. Now you are embarrassed to leave the house.

> *My wife hated to go out with our son because they were both covered with formula half the time. One day I bought us all matching grey sweat suits that don't show the spit-up. I also got her a bottle of perfume. I don't think she really appreciated this.*

Maybe you are worried that people will think you are an incompetent parent and don't know how to take care of your child. Maybe you feel that you really aren't a good enough parent and you are afraid people will spot you are just pretending to be a good parent.

Maybe you hate to ask for help. The most independent people can have the most trouble asking for help when they need it.

> *I volunteer at our church and at my son's school all the time. I'm the one that people call when they need help. There is no way that I'm going to call and ask for help. I would much rather do it all myself than admit I'm not a perfect parent.*

You may be very embarrassed about your financial situation. It may the first time you have not had enough money to cover the bills and this new experience can be scary. Or the financial situation may have already been pretty bad and caring for your baby with reflux may make a bad situation a whole lot worse. Many mothers can't go back to work because their baby requires too much care and too many doctor's appointments.

Tight finances can cause more embarrassment when you can't pay a baby sitter, you can't have any help with the cleaning or the lawn, bill collectors are calling and you are reluctant to take your baby to the doctor when she needs to go because you can't pay the bill.

Denial

We hear a lot of complaints from mothers that fathers and grandparents just don't want to believe anything is wrong with the baby. Many people use denial as a way of avoiding the problem – if you don't acknowledge that there even is a problem, then you don't have to fix it or find somebody to blame for it. It can be a warped way of trying to keep the peace – by pretending everything is fine.

Fathers were often raised to be "tough" and ignore health problems. Researchers have documented time after time that many men don't even go to the emergency room when they have chest pain. This attitude carries over to ignoring health problems in their kids.

I used to be the King of Denial. I did not believe for a minute that anything was wrong with my son that firm parenting couldn't fix. My wife finally forced my mother and I to go with her to see the pediatrician. He told us in no uncertain terms that our baby was in significant pain and that his refusal to eat really was a big deal. He also helped me see that ignoring my son's illness meant that I was calling my wife a liar.

I guess I'm a little bit in denial - I keep thinking that she doesn't REALLY have reflux, and that giving her all this medicine is totally unnecessary. Just yesterday, I was telling somebody what a waste of time this is – I guess it is karma that the baby puked all over me this morning and has been crying for hours.

Confused

Learning how to take care of a baby with reflux can make your head spin. About medical treatment decisions, about mixed messages from doctors, about mixed messages from friends/family. More…

I know something needs to be done – but what? Today, I want to ask the doctor to change her meds, her formula, I want to buy her a hammock bed and get a new sling and try letting her cry it out. If I did all this in one day, my poor baby would be a mess and so would I. And if something worked, we would never know which thing helped. I'm so confused.

My daughter had reflux many years ago and recently she had leukemia. In some ways, dealing with the leukemia was simpler. The doctors all agreed on what to do about the leukemia. But the reflux treatment was long, confusing, contradictory, contentious and not particularly successful.

Today, I gave the medicine to the wrong twin. I got hysterical and called poison control. I don't know why I thought it is safe for one of the twins but somehow thought it would be dangerous for the other twin. I'm so out of it I worry I might do something more dangerous.

Insecure

When your baby cries all the time and you can't make her stop, you can start to feel like you aren't a good mother. When you feed her the best you can but she still doesn't gain weight well enough, you can start to feel that you don't know what you are doing. When she thrashes in your arms and you don't know what to do, it is hard to feel competent. When you are used to fixing problems and this one just defies your efforts to solve it, you can start to feel very insecure.

I normally have strong opinions and research everything. I feel like a rubber toy being pushed and pulled everywhere. I normally know exactly what needs to be done, but not now. All I want to do is help my baby feel better and I'm completely clueless how to do this.

Depressed

Some mothers suffer from severe hormone swings after their baby is born and these hormone swings can keep you dwelling on negative issues. It can take a year for a new mother's hormones to level out and you may be more prone to tears and self-criticism during this time.

It is well documented that mothers of babies with 'severe colic' are much more likely to become depressed. If you find that negative thoughts are interfering with doing what needs to be done, it may be a signal to seek help. Taking care of a baby with reflux is challenging and this type of stress can tip the baby blues into full-blown post partum depression.

Most people don't realize that post partum depression can be VERY serious. Some women get so confused that they hallucinate. If you feel yourself losing your grip, talk to friends, your family and your doctor about your difficulties. The bottom line is you need to take care of yourself so that you can take care of your baby.

FamilyDoctor.org lists the following symptoms of postpartum depression:
> Loss of interest or pleasure in life
> Loss of appetite
> Less energy and motivation to do things
> A hard time falling asleep or staying asleep
> Sleeping more than usual
> Increased crying or tearfulness
> Feeling worthless, hopeless or overly guilty
> Feeling restless, irritable or anxious
> Unexplained weight loss or gain
> Feeling like life isn't worth living
> Having thoughts about hurting yourself
> Worrying about hurting your baby

Bringing in the Professionals: When to Seek Counseling

Reflux is extremely stressful. You can get emotional support and companionship from other parents of children with reflux but sometimes is it is also helpful to talk with a counselor or physician. Marriage counseling or individual counseling may be a positive step toward coping with the stress of intensive care parenting.

Your family, especially your children, are counting on you to be available to them. It is important for you to get the support and assistance that you need so you can keep helping them.

If you seek counseling, try to find a professional who is knowledgeable about the impact of illness on families. You certainly don't want one more person telling you to let the baby cry-it-out.

> It does help to talk to someone professionally like a counselor. I finally did when my daughter was 15 months and I wish I had done it from day one. I am still over-reactive at times about things. That only gets better with time and as your child starts to age and you feel like the reflux is getting more manageable. After 15 months of depression and fear, I have finally climbed out of the isolation and darkness to see that it is going to be OK. It may be different, but eventually it will be OK, and maybe even better.

> I was so depressed and anxious that at 9 weeks I finally went to my doctor and got help. I got on medication for 6 months and it really did take the edge off and let me get much needed naps when she did actually nap. If you think it might help...run, don't walk, to your doctor. Reflux is SO stressful on the entire family, you have to do whatever it takes to hold yourself together until your family gets past it.

> Depressed? You bet. Caring for the constantly crying "Love of my life" 24-7 alone (hubby was out of state) certainly took its toll - on my body, my sleep patterns, and eventually my mind. I felt extremely unsupported and alone, endlessly pacing the floors with my new bundle of "joy". Why didn't I seek help?

During a support group meeting, one mom said she was considering taking anti-depressants and wanted to know how common this was. Many of the moms felt that this should be standard practice for all! It is very common for mothers of refluxers to suffer from some degree of sleep deprivation, anxiety, depression, isolation, etc., from caring for such sick and uncomfortable children. If we were issued round-the-clock nurses and housekeepers things would be a lot easier. But this is the real deal and it often comes down to one very tired mom doing way too much day after day (and night after night).

Reflux Parent's Lament

As I pace the floor at three a.m.,
I don't understand, I can't comprehend,

Why my baby's awake and crying again,
My heart aches for this child I love so dearly,
A few hours' sleep and I'd see things more clearly,
I'd climb to the stars and reach to the sky,
If somewhere, somehow, I'd find the answer why.
I search back in my memory for something I've done,
To cause such pain and misery to my dear little one.
When feeling well she's the light of our lives,
When the pain comes upon her,
Her screams cut through us like knives.
She looks so well, family and friends don't understand,
Our family is crumbling; we could sure use a hand.
Tests, medications, doctor's visits galore,
I know other mothers sure find me a bore.
We're impatient and angry and very confused,
It's hard to explain - even the doctors aren't sure,
The prognosis for reflux just seems so obscure.
We'd do anything to help her, we hope and we pray,
But for now, we just try to get by day to day.
I know for sure we'll lick this thing in the end,
And soon our sweet baby will be on the mend.

Anonymous

Coping Tips

Surviving day to day may seem challenging but it is possible to get by.
We hope these parent-tested and strategies will help you.

Teamwork

It is time to mobilize TEAM REFLUX! You and your family need to
form a strong parenting team. Remember the key to teamwork is communicating often and expressing wants and needs. It is everyone's re-
sponsibility to listen carefully and acknowledge feelings and needs.

> *Sometimes I had to give my husband a big hint that I needed help. I
> would say, "If you want dinner, come home 30 minutes before you
> are hungry!" With three children under the age of five, this was nei-
> ther a joke nor a threat. My husband would come in the door and
> corral the kids while I headed for the kitchen to make a quick meal. I
> would turn on the radio, sip a bit of wine and get the food on the ta-*

ble. By working together as a team, we were able to have a real dinner several nights a week.

While it is easy to blame the other parent and put up a wall of anger, it will do little to help the situation. The whole family needs to develop a plan, work together and support each other's efforts.

My husband just didn't understand how hard it is to care for a baby with reflux. Two things made a difference – I left him completely alone with her for a full day and I made a list of the fifty zillion tasks I perform each day for her and the family. It helped him understand why I couldn't just take it all in stride like his mother did when she raised five boys. Her kids entertained themselves in the neighborhood – she didn't have carpool, soccer and play dates and they ate meatloaf with potatoes every night. She didn't even have a list.

Next week, I'm planning to ask him to take five things off my list and put them on his. I also scratched my name off the top of my list and scribbled in a new title – Stuff That Has to Get Done and Nobody Else is Willing to Do. It isn't really 'my' list and calling it 'my' list lets my husband off the hook. We had a pretty heated talk about this before he realized it was unfair.

Second Shift

Even Team Reflux needs a second shift. Sometimes the job is too big for two parents. You may find that there is a need for an additional adult to help with the household and the baby. It is surprising how tolerant another adult is to a crying baby as long as they get to go home at the end of the day.

Some parents find that they need to take care of the baby because no one else can manage the feeding and the comforting. They ask their helpers to do chores and errands. Others find that they like a break from the care giving.

If someone offers to watch the kids, make hot meal, run to the store or vacuum, this is the time to accept all offers. When this phase of your life is over, you can return the favor for someone else.

My parents came to stay with us after another tearful phone call about how hard it was to take care of my daughter. They came in and immediately rolled up their sleeves and helped us in so many ways - shopping, rocking the baby, making meals, etc. Within a week, THEY were on the brink of exhaustion and called a nanny agency to hire a full-time caregiver. It took five adults to take care of one little baby!

If you feel you can't leave anybody else in charge and leave the house, get somebody to be there with you. They can help you out and keep you company at the same time. It used to be common to hire a *mother's helper* just to have another pair of hands during the day. A *dula* is the current term for somebody who takes care of the mom and the house so mom can take care of the baby.

Take Care of Yourself

This seems like such a cliché. When no one but you can calm the baby or keep the milk from urping up, how are you supposed to take a break? Of course you would love a break but who is going to take over? You are still waiting for Mary Poppins to appear at your door.

Everyone says, take some time to do what you enjoy, read a book, go out to eat. You are happy just to take a shower and chew your food. You don't even know what day of the week it is much less what book is on the best sellers list.

Try to do something little, something symbolic. Perhaps you will sit at the table and eat rather than standing at the counter eating and writing out the bills while on hold with the doctor's office.

Take your vitamins, eat well, and maintain your own health. It is surprising how something as little as drinking enough water during the day can provide more energy and balance. Find a way to get a bit of exercise. Even if you have to exercise with your baby attached to you. It is hard work. But remember, you are the most important person in the world to your baby and she needs you to stay healthy and well.

I tried to take a walk every day. I think she felt better when we went outside for a walk either in the sling or in the stroller. It was a change of pace and felt good for both of us. An added benefit is that the house didn't get messier by the minute when we weren't in it!

I've been so tired from lack of sleep at night and trying to soothe her all day that I've actually been sick a few times. Ordinarily I'm a very healthy person. Now, I feel like I catch every bug that comes along.

Caregiver Routine

Taking care of a baby with reflux is like running a marathon. You need to pace yourself. As much as possible, develop a schedule. It is likely that a schedule will help you feel more in control and will help your baby feel more settled too. Naturally, there will be days when you will need to abandon your schedule and just do what needs to be done.

Every afternoon at 4pm the crying would start. And just about every afternoon, I would place my son in the stroller and headed up the street. Everyone could hear the wailing as we passed. Before long, a neighbor or two would stop to say hello or join me on the walk. It became a bit of a joke-everyone knew we were coming from a mile away since he was so noisy!

I would not say that we had a routine for the day; it was more like a rhythm. It helped me as much as it helped my daughter. At sun up, it was time to eat breakfast. Before lunch, we always took a walk. After lunch was time to nap. When my husband came home, I took a few minutes to be alone or complete a task without interruption. After dinner was bath and rocking time before bed.

My story: I'm not a routine person at all. I raised my first child to be as flexible as I could. He could sleep anywhere at any time and eat anything put in front of him. Katie just wasn't the same. She really benefited from being on more of a schedule. If she skipped a nap, she was a mess and her reflux would act up. If meals were late, it seemed to bother her tummy.

Trust your Instincts

Go ahead, trust your instincts. Go with your gut. Hear your inner voice. You are an expert on your child. You know what is best for her. It isn't just intuition, you are with her more hours of every day and there is no way that anybody else can "read" her as well as you can.

Surround yourself with people who know you and care about you. Confide in those who value your opinion and support your decisions.

A few years ago, PAGER Association collaborated with TAP Pharmaceutical Products, Inc on a pediatric reflux awareness campaign, Gut Instincts, When You Know Something is Wrong with Your Child. Parents of refluxers often use the phrase "go with your gut" or "trust your gut" to encourage another parent to seek help for their baby.

Let Go of Other Responsibilities

It may seem like there are too many items on the "TO DO" list and you are falling hopelessly behind. You never get anything crossed off the list and more items are added daily.

It is time to take a good hard look at your responsibilities and decide what really needs to be done: taking care of the baby, eating, sleeping.

That may be all you keep on the list. Remember, this is a season in parenting - it is a time of intensive care parenting because you have a child who needs you more than anything else. Eventually, this season will end and she will not be little forever.

> I thought my husband was getting upset about our messy house and seldom getting dinner on the table. When we talked, I was surprised that he didn't care half as much as I thought. He agreed that my sanity was more important.

Live in the Present Tense

Living in the present tense means focusing on the moment you are in. Look at where you are, what you are doing. Put all of your energy into that moment. It is easy for caretakers to multi-task. You are reading the picture book while planning dinner and remembering to call the refill in to the pharmacy. Clear your head and focus on the book, your child, your closeness to each other. Smell the sweetness of her hair, feel the closeness and relaxation you both feel. You are living in the present.

> I always carry a notebook with me that has my ToDo list. When the list would get so ridiculously long that I didn't have a prayer of putting a dent in it, I would just put a rubber band around the book sealing it shut and attach a big note to the cover – "Have Some Fun with the Kids."

Network

Several studies show that patients and families who develop a network of support through a patient support group or organization have a better medical outcome than those who do not seek information.

> Before I contacted PAGER Association, I felt very isolated and frustrated. I searched everywhere for patient information and only came across books about adults with acid reflux. Even though I had wonderful doctors and a supportive family, I still needed to speak to other parent. It was a powerful experience to actually talk with someone who understood what I was talking about and I felt empowered to try new treatments and have a positive outlook on the situation.

Parent-to-parent networking such as an online forum or chat group allows parents to post messages, vent, ask questions and share ideas.

> Posted: I'm so glad your daughter is doing better. We were all worried about her and you. You WILL GET THROUGH THIS. Somehow, someway. And soon you'll be here helping someone else going through the exact same thing.

> Posted: I don't feel so alone in this anymore. It is so nice to meet people who "get it." Doesn't it feel good to know that someone else is in the same situation? I know it makes me feel much better. After awhile, you realize that it's no use talking to friends because they just don't get it. I was never criticized like some of you, but I haven't gotten any support, much less sympathy, from people who haven't been here. Good meaning people will make remarks like: all babies cry a lot, you know. My baby doesn't cry - she SCREAMS - and it's not normal. Even when they are trying to be supportive and kind, they aren't very effective.

> Posted: Even though I haven't been able to post much, just reading other posts helps me stay sane. I cried when I read your posting, I was there! We still struggle with reflux, but for us it is getting so much better (though three weeks ago, I didn't know if I'd ever sleep again). As I was reading your posting, I thought of my own low point several months ago, venting on this board and being uplifted by all

the kind, thoughtful, hopeful responses. I am so grateful I found this board -- can you imagine how much MORE isolated we'd all be fifteen years ago, before the internet, before this means of communicating existed? Anyway, I just wanted you to know I hurt for you and really hope things get better.

Posted: Hang in there and know many of us have walked in your sleep deprived shoes and survived to smile and laugh again. The thing is - you WILL get through this. You really will - I promise. You actually have no choice. The bad thing is that it is not going to be easy and there are going to be lots of days when you are going minute-to-minute, and just trying to get through the day. You will feel so many different emotions at once - how can you actually love your baby so deeply but at the exact same time almost hate them for what is happening? It's hard to remember at times, but it's not the baby's fault - it's the reflux's fault. Your son is in a lot of pain and is scared. And even though there's not all that much you can do a lot of the time, just being there for him to cry on is enough it seems.

♦

Posted: I stumbled upon your website, I am so glad I found you. I've been reading the posts for quite some time now, looking to feel less isolated with the struggles that go along with parenting sick kids. It's been helping and I am impressed by the supportive community available here.

Humor

Having a baby with reflux may not seem funny, but sometimes, you just have to laugh. Otherwise, you will end up crying or feeling angry. At PAGER Association, we have heard some hilarious stories. Sometimes you just have to laugh!

I'm pretty sure I hold the world record for paying for puke. During the pre holiday rush, I took my infant son food shopping despite the risks involved. My son is a champion spitter and can cover a car seat, freshly laundered clothes and carpeting in no time. Things were going pretty well until we got to the produce section. Before you could say Brussel sprouts, he had managed to vomit into a bag of fresh, ripe pears! I am a veteran reflux mom and I had dealt with my share of reflux emergencies so I knew just what to do. I simply put the messy bag of pears in the cart and proceeded to the check-

out. The clerk raised the bag of pears onto the scale and said, "Ma'am, there's something wrong with the pears. Do you want to get some new ones?" I calmly said, "It's OK.. My son vomited into the bag." So the clerk weighed the pears, plus goo and sent us on our way, leaving a few bemused shoppers in line.

My story: One of my coping methods has been to find the humor when telling my friends about the crisis-of-the-day. When I went to the pediatrician (almost every week!), I would do a short comedy routine for the staff when they asked, "How was your week?" I wrote down many of the stories in a journal. Usually, I didn't have time to write them out fully, but I would make a couple of quick notes and I wrote them into full stories years later. The kids love to read stories about the crazy things they did.

Celebrate This Child

So by now you have thrown out the parenting books and the rulebook about how you are supposed to raise children. It is time to look beyond the worry and the stress and take a good look at this child. Celebrate who she is. Focus on her beautiful little body, her warm, smooth skin, hers little nose that looks like Aunt Mary's. Take pictures of her. How about a picture of her finally falling asleep on dad's shoulder (notice that dad is asleep too!) or crying in Grandma's arms. Maybe you couldn't take a picture of her actually eating cake on her first birthday. Go ahead and take a picture of her anyway with her cute outfit and party hat. Be quick.

Dealing with Advice from Others

You may begin to doubt yourself when family, friends, doctors and strangers give you well- meaning advice. You may be told, "Let her cry it out," "All babies eat when they are hungry," "You are spoiling her by holding her all of the time," "She will never learn to sleep in her crib if you keep taking her into your bed." Normally, you would just take these comments in stride. However, at the moment, you are in no mood for advice and unsolicited judgment of your parenting decisions.

People just can't hold back from giving advice to parents. From friends and relatives to total strangers, everyone has something to say. Advice on eating and sleeping seems to be favorite topics. You may feel as if you will have a temper tantrum every time someone makes a comment or gives a tidbit of advice. While the comments are well meaning, they seem to de-value your parenting and lead to self-doubt and confusion.

Ideas for dealing with advice:

One sentence explanation: Have a short explanation for your child's issues-she is crying because of the acid reflux.

Refrain from commenting: You do not have to agree or disagree with what other people say. Just change the topic, pretend you didn't hear or walk away.

Find a circle of support: Find a friend or support group and share your feelings in a safe environment.

Quote the doctor: The doctor said, "She needs to be held most of the time."

On line chat/support group: Use the internet to find others for a virtual support group.

Humor: don't take the advice too seriously. Use humor to respond to comments.

Look on the Bright Side

As difficult as the journey has been, many parents report that dealing with reflux has given them a new outlook at life.

I don't take anything for granted.
I take one thing at a time.
I don't worry about the little stuff as much.
I have a special bond with my child since we spent so much time together.
I can read her like a book.
I have met new friends.
I have received support and help from others and that has given me hope.
I have helped her get well.
We have weathered the storm together.

Notes:

12 Family and Caregiver Issues

While there is a lot of focus on the impact of reflux on moms, in reality, reflux affects the whole family. Dads, siblings and grandparents all feel strong emotions such as frustration, confusion and exhaustion.

> *Life has been very challenging since my son was born. I have a very strong relationship with my husband and we have a lot of love for each other. I've managed not to get upset (much) at him by reminding myself that it's not him I resent, but the situation. The same goes for my son. I love him, but hate our situation. It's been very hard for me to watch my husband do normal things like shower every day and change his clothes. He doesn't have to sit in shirts that smell like old breast milk or deal with hairy legs for weeks on end.*

The way we deal with health issues depends on our parenting styles, our perception of our role and how we deal with stress. It is important to recognize that our concerns and coping styles may clash with those around us during a health care crisis.

Many of the personality style issues from the chapter about working with the medical team apply to the family dynamics. All the things that affect how you work with the medical team affect how members of your family work as a team – your experiences with the medical profession, your perception of illness and your confidence level all play a role in family dynamics.

One thing that stress tends to do to family members is to magnify their personalities. A person who tends to be a bit of an avoider, will want to run away in the face of this horrible medical situation. The person who likes to become an expert during a small crisis might start to be overbearing as the crisis becomes larger. Somebody who is very defensive and insecure may act more stubborn. And the person who tends to get angry may feel they would like nothing better than to throw a tantrum in the face of the stress.

As adults who are in charge of caring for a sick child, you owe it to your child to stop and think about how you really want to act during this crisis instead of doing what comes naturally. Is your baby going to get the care she needs if you run away, become too bossy, dig in your heels or act hostile? The stress from reflux can make you stronger and it can make your whole family stronger if you all pull together to help your baby – even if that means learning how you react to stress and slowly changing to a more constructive pattern.

People in your family can be going through different coping stages at different times and to different degrees. You might be mildly mourning the loss of the perfect infancy you planned for, your spouse may be angry and frustrated and your mother-in-law my be very deeply in denial all at the same time. You may all go through variations of the other stages but at such different times that it seems you are all on completely different wavelengths.

> *During the worst of reflux (0-4 months), I felt like I was a "single married mother" because my husband was going through the "adjustment and denial" period. I did not have time to go through the adjustment period - I had a refluxer on my hands, and had it not been for my Mom and this board, I would probably have gone to the very depths of depression.*

Relatives who don't every get to experience the 'joy' of a whole day with your baby can't possibly understand all that you go through. Unless they have been the sole caretaker for a miserable baby who screams constantly, can't sleep and won't eat, they can't really know what you are going through.

> *They just don't get it. They end up making me feel like it's my fault she won't eat. If I react the way I want to, I'll end up starting a family brawl on Christmas.*

What Dads Want

Because mom is usually the one who spends more time with the baby, she is often viewed as the expert. Dads often get left out of caretaking and it may seem that only mom can take care of this baby. Most dads want to have a turn with feeding, bathing and diapering. Remember how long it took you to be able to do this without jostling the baby and provoking a reflux episode? Give him some space to practice.

Mom might use soothing methods when the baby is unhappy, but Dad might choose to use distraction - and it might work better for him. Even babies react differently in the same situation depending on what adults are around them.

> *My wife was completely thrilled to discover that our son will take a bottle of breast milk from me. There is no way on earth she can convince him to take a bottle because he knows that she has the real deal and gets upset. It is hard to believe a tiny baby knows which one of us has the breasts. I'm a bit jealous that she always seems to know what he wants and I don't feel like I have a clue most of the time. This my turn to do something she can't.*

Mom wants to talk about her day, her long night, and her fears. Dad may be focused on the finances and earning a living. Neither is wrong and neither can read the other's mind. Everyone needs to communicate clearly and frequently.

> *One thing that really helped us was to both read some of the postings on reflux.org. We were both in tears when we read about the problems that some other couples are having. It gave us a chance to talk things out. It turns out we were both extremely worried but we show it differently.*

There might be times when there isn't any clear or right course of action. It is quite natural for one parent to be in favor of one idea and the other parent to favor a different option. Each of you need to calmly discuss the pros and cons of each option.

> *When we are facing a decision about changing treatment, my hubby likes to play "devil's advocate" and try to think of all the things that can go wrong. I finally told him that this might be a great skill at work, but it makes me want to strangle him because it comes across as extremely negative at a time when I'm desperate for reassurance and hope.*

Sometimes Dad finds it easier to be assertive with others who care for your baby.

> My darling hubby and I had a great conversation on the way to one of our earlier appointments with our Ped GI. He said, 'If they blow us off, then I'm going to ask him how much he makes per hour and tell him we're hiring him for the day to come to our house, live our life and witness our baby's quality of life and then they WILL do something for him.' My hero!

Dad needs to hear some positive words, from you. "Thank you, it was nice to have a break." "You are doing a good job." "The baby likes it when you do that." Dads also need to remember that Mom needs to hear your positive feedback as well. Your positive attitude and kind words will make her day!

> I insisted we change my son's meds thinking it would help him more. Well he was horrible on the new stuff. I felt so bad for him. I felt I had done something to hurt him. My wife reminded me that I was only trying to take good care of our baby and that I am a good dad. It made me feel better.

Mom needs a nap and a break from the baby. Guess what? Dad needs some downtime too. It is important to communicate these needs and have a coordinated approach so everybody in the house gets a break.

> Our baby will only nap on my chest. I have more padding than my wife does and I can sit a lot stiller than she can. The baby naps for hours while I watch TV. I am also the champion baby burper. Of course.

Dad misses the old days when he had your full attention. Parenting decreases the amount of 'couples' time. Parenting a child with reflux might bring this down to mere minutes each day. Try to make the most of those precious minutes.

> I know it has been hard on my wife, caring for our son with reflux. He takes a lot of her time and energy. I try to help as much as I can. I know my wife loves me and I appreciate what she does, but I miss spending time alone with her. I don't think our lack of private time bothers her nearly as much as it bothers me.

Try to be creative and find some time together. You might be surprised at how 15 minutes of "in-tune-with-each-other-time" can help. It may take several tries but you need a little time alone regularly.

> *When my hubby and I were desperate for some alone time, we would go to Starbucks for an hour. We pay 6 dollars for coffee and 7 dollars for the hour of babysitting. But hey, a date for 13 bucks isn't bad! Getting out in the evening was too stressful and trying to find a sitter for a baby who cries all evening is impossible. These breakfast and coffee dates are saving our marriage. We call it speed dating.*

Some Dads were raised to be tough at all times. Having a sick child might be the experience that lets Dad be more tender than he might be otherwise.

> *I'm a big guy but my little daughter has me wrapped around her little finger. My wife has somehow gotten used to the constant crying, but I don't think I ever will. It breaks my heart and pierces my eardrums.*

Mothers may get all of the sympathy and support even though dads may be just as disappointed/worried and stressed as mom. Many men feel completely comfortable expressing their fears and worries, but some need encouragement.

Dads who are used to being in charge, might have a harder time coping with an illness that they can't "fix." This can be particularly hard for Dads who are normally in charge at their jobs. They often like concrete ways of making progress.

> *I was too busy to get on the computer so my husband sat down and did some research on reflux. It made him feel good to have a meaningful job to do and he learned that all of the reflux moms on the discussion boards sounded just as worn out as his wife!!!*

Cautionary Tales - What Moms need Dads to Know

Often, moms get very frustrated and angry with Dads. They may be jealous of the fact that fathers get to have a life outside the house. They may resent when a father doesn't participate in caring for the sick child. They may be terrified that reflux will destroy their marriage. They may feel that Dad should support them more when the relatives or doctors don't give the help they need.

I think my husband can't bear the problems with our son since he can't "fix" them so he just withdraws instead. This has been a tremendous burden on me. He doesn't take the time to understand our son's medical problems so he really can't help with finding solutions. Do I feel resentful because of this? YES! It is extremely lonely, scary and frustrating when you are trying to deal with a reflux baby all alone. As if it isn't bad enough that you have to encounter less-than-helpful doctor's, well-meaning but undereducated friends, relatives and in-laws, but then to not have the full and total support of your husband? It is almost too much to bear sometimes. As a matter of fact, my husband did not even really believe our HAD reflux until about 3 months ago. He believed the doctor's diagnosis of "colic." His lack of trust in me was seriously damaging to our relationship.

My husband can't be bothered to take care of his own health. He completely denies that he has serious reflux. I don't know what made me think he would take his son's health more seriously.

At this point, I've given up on my husband or his family accepting that my baby has reflux. I found a great doctor and he is my other team member. I don't even bother telling my husband about the appointments anymore. We have been at one doctor or another every week.

In my husband's family, a dirty car is completely unacceptable. I have been trying to convince him that the car is not important right now. If he doesn't get in the house and help with the baby, he will be living in that car.

What Grandparents and Extended Family Want

Grandparents feel a deep connection and bond to their grandchildren. So it makes sense that they may experience a high level of anxiety and fear about an illness that affects their grandchild.

Unfortunately, when you are all stressed and worried, communication may break down and attempts to help might make the situation worse. That is why some parents feel the grandparents are meddling when they attempt to give advice, help with the chores or call their golf partner who is a pediatrician.

> *I was already feeling like a bad mother and when my mother and mother-in-law give me advice, it just made me feel worse. I just wanted so much to feel in charge and feel like an adult. I couldn't find a way to say that I wanted sympathy and support but not advice.*

Grandparents want to fix the problem affecting their precious grandchild and help you too. Remember, you are always the child in the eyes of your parents and they want to kiss the hurts and offer hugs for the disappointment.

Grandparents may need to be educated about new approaches to treatment. In the past, parents were instructed to let their fussy babies cry it out so they would not get spoiled. You may believe very strongly that crying it out is bad, but they were told just as strongly that it was right and it might take a bit of time to adjust to the current mindset. Research that wasn't available when they were raising you shows letting a baby cry in pain is harmful.

> *My mother had a really hard time with the concept of not letting a baby cry in pain. She had her babies in an era when picking up a crying baby was equal to letting your toddler sass you – it was a sign of weak parenting. One day we had a real heart-to-heart talk about crying and babies who feel pain. I suddenly realized that she was holding strong to her beliefs because admitting that hurting babies need to be picked up would mean admitting that she had been cruel to me when I was a baby and had reflux. At that moment, I understood why she was clinging to the cry-it-out thing.*

> *When my baby with reflux got to be a toddler and she still wasn't putting herself to sleep, we had another discussion. My mother said that some children need to be rocked but others just seem to need to cry before they can fall asleep. She was right. After about three minutes of crying (not shrieking), my toddler fell right asleep. Mom was right in this case.*

When your parents were raising you, if a baby was really fussy or the mother was hysterical and exhausted, mom or baby might have been offered sedation or sleeping pills.

A few months after my daughter was born, I was leafing through my baby book. I came across a prescription that had been taped into the book. My mom said that I had been a fussy baby and the doctor prescribed a strong sedative for me. She never filled it because she didn't see how sedating me was going to take care of my pain.

On the other hand, grandma may be more patient than you are when it comes to walking a fussy baby back and forth across the room for hours on end.

I had never heard of the colic hold. My mother-in-law demonstrated this odd way of holding a fussy baby. It looked so strange, but it actually worked quite well.

◆

Katie's Grandma says: My dentist taught me the ultimate fussy baby trick. My granddaughter only wanted her Mommy to hold her and would cry inconsolably when I tried to baby-sit. I got one of Beth's lightly worn T-shirts out of the laundry pile and put it on. Suddenly, Katie decided I smelled right and let me hold her.

Personality differences are often magnified during any crisis situation. Somebody who is passive, might get more passive and nearly give up. Somebody who tends to get frustrated, might become very angry. A person who tends to look for somebody to blame when things go wrong is even more likely to do this during a crisis. What bugs you now, may turn into a major personality clash during tough times.

My grandmother is a wonderful human being, but she can drive me a bit crazy. She is a huge worrier and gets very flustered in a crisis. Right after my baby was diagnosed, she drove me nuts. She got all worked up and worried that the baby was going to choke or die in her sleep. I just blew up. I told her I needed her to be calm so that I could be the one to freak out. I was just raving, but deep down it made some twisted sense.

One issue that often causes trouble in families is when toddlers with reflux misbehave because they are in pain.

Cautionary Tales for Family and Friends

My mother-in-law kept telling my husband and me that my daughter's symptoms were psychosomatic and that we were giving her too much attention for a made-up illness! I no longer speak to my in-laws much and when they ask about my daughter's health, I always say, "She's fine." We no longer include them in the loop when it comes to medical issues. They obviously don't really want to know the truth, so we don't tell them the truth.

I will never forgive my In-laws for not supporting us. We don't really speak to them anymore. I'm glad that you can forgive your parents, but maybe you are a better person than me, or maybe you didn't have quite the reflux hell that I went through, or maybe your parents weren't quite as condescending, critical, and uncaring as my in-laws were. They saw exactly what was wrong with my daughter but they still thought I was a hypochondriac. My parents helped us SOOOOOOOO much. I would have drowned without them. They got me to the doctors and got me on antidepressants eventually so that I could cope - that is how much stress I was under. During that time, all my in-laws would do would be to come over for 20 minutes, hold the baby, look at her and wonder why she was crying so much, tell us we weren't feeding her the right formula and we needed to see another doctor, and then leave. Later they would call my husband and ask why I was so rude to them - uh, because I hadn't slept since she was born!!!! Three months before!!! And hadn't showered in a week!!! Or eaten in two days!

One night we had to run to the hospital with our older child. We asked two different relatives to take our gerdling and neither would do it. A dear friend took her and said, "Don't come get her till morning - you need to sleep." It still makes me angry at times that the family was not supportive. But when I think of all the times my husband and I played "pass the baby before she goes out the window" I guess I understand.

I went through a very dark period where I really started to believe that my son would be better off without me because the relatives thought I was crazy. I've had to learn (the hard way!) that a mother's

instinct is SO strong and your gut will tell you when your child needs help or is in pain. I try not to listen to those who doubt the way we are treating our son, even though sometimes it's so hard. No one can really understand except the other parents who have been through this.

Don't waste your breath trying to convince people. You need that precious energy for helping your daughter. I only get emotional with the people who HAVE been there for us. I feel like life is so fleeting now, and I truly believe that God puts people on earth to help you through.(I'm not religious really, but with our reflux journey, we continually get help exactly when we feel like we no longer can take it one more second.) I let people know how very much I appreciate them. If I didn't tell them, they'd never know how that one chat, or that one dinner, or that one day babysitting helped save my sanity during those early months. And they should know so they can tell others if they hear of other kids with reflux. I'm sure our specialists think I need medication because of the sappy letters I write all the time after we visit and they get my baby back on track!

My mother, mother-in-law and older relatives are constantly asking "how I know" it's reflux in my 9 month old. They honestly think this is a "fake" disease that our pediatrician is making up. They say "all babies spit-up and he barely even does that." (He's a silent refluxer now that he's on meds.) I try to explain his painful crying (which they say all babies cry), his back arching (I get a blank stare on that one that says "so?"), his sleeplessness (to which they say "babies aren't supposed to sleep right"), to I can HEAR when it comes up, he coughs and chokes then cries (yet another blank stare for that). Finally, I explain he stops all symptoms for at least a while medicated and he's finally happy - and they still don't get it. Does anyone else encounter this from the older generation? ("babies never had reflux when I had kids...") So then, they try to make me feel bad for giving him prescription meds (which I already hate doing, but I have to or else he's miserable).

What Siblings Want

Having a sick baby in the house is very difficult for siblings, too. Even siblings who are too young to really understand what is going on.

The good news is that your child will probably grow up to be insightful and more sympathetic than his peers. The bad news is that things may be a bit rocky at times.

Older brothers and sisters often feel concern about a sick sibling. All of those urgent phone calls and sudden trips to the hospital combined with one look at your worried face is all they need to think the worse.

Children don't always thing logically. They may think it was their fault the baby is sick, or they may think that the baby is going to die. They may think that the doctors are causing the baby's pain or that the baby has been bad and is being punished. They may even think reflux is contagious.

Some siblings deal with stress by being as helpful as they can be. Like a little adult. It may seem sweet at first, but it is not a great family dynamic to encourage. They may be engaging in "magical thinking" and believe that their sibling's medical problems will get better if they display "perfect" behavior.

Acting perfect takes an emotional toll and can make them feel guilty if they are less than perfect and then the baby happens to feel worse the next day.

Kids who skip the usual self-centered, carefree and irresponsible behavior that all kids go through might display these behaviors much later when the crisis is over – possibly at an age when it isn't socially acceptable to act childish.

Other children take out their anger and frustration by reverting to an old pattern of behavior (having potty accidents) or acting out (emptying the flour on the kitchen floor while you are cleaning vomit off the couch). They don't know they are doing this – it is all subconscious and punishment doesn't help. Older children may fall in with a bad crowd and not have any realization they are doing it so you will pay attention to them.

When the drama of reflux is over, you may find that another sibling issue comes to light. Some children are so used to the drama that they feel very uneasy when the house is calm and running smoothly. This feels so strange to them that they might subconsciously cause new drama.

Practical Ideas for Siblings

Stick to a routine as much as possible. When the whole world feels out of sync, routine is particularly important.

Schedule one-to-one parent time for a story, a few minutes on the swing or other activity. It may be simpler to hand off the sibling to other caregivers, but remember to keep some of the sibling time for yourself and hand off the baby.

The siblings want to be part of TEAM REFLUX too. Let them help you care for the baby but don't put pressure on them to be too responsible. Ask them to help with simple tasks, but make it clear that big jobs like giving medicine are for adults only.

> *My story: My three year old unhooked the real baby from her baby monitor and hooked up a doll. He told us that "his" baby was sick, too. So we gave him a vital job as the in-home Spit Up Alert System. Whenever the baby vomited, he yelled, "Blurp Alert!!" at the top of his lungs.*

Ask your child what questions she has about the illness so that you can give her correct information. Tummy Trouble is a rhyming book about a bunny with reflux. And let your older child know that you want her to come to you when she has questions.

> *We were trying to shelter our son by not talking about the medical situation in front of him. Apparently, he thought this meant things were even worse than they were and his imagination was working overtime. Now, when there is a new development, we give him a one-sentence summary.*

Give your older child permission to express her needs and concerns to you. When she is young, you might have to help her find the words to express what they feel. She may resent all the time you spend with the sick child. She may resent the financial burden and not being able to buy things or go places. She may feel that the sick sibling is getting special treatment and doesn't get punished as much. She may be embarrassed by all the drama or they may feel guilty for being healthy.

> *I tell my daughter, "You must be disappointed that we have to bring the baby to the doctor instead of going to the park. I wish we could go to the park too." I let her express anger at the new baby to grown-ups and I never tell her that her anger is wrong, but make I it clear that she can never act out her anger toward the baby.*

Often children will express themselves using pictures or stories.

> *My big girl came home from preschool with a picture titled My Family. There was the baby all snug between mom and dad in the middle of the picture. My older daughter was playing by herself in the corner. I could see that she felt small, left out and alone.*

Thank your child for being understanding and patient. You can also let her overhear you telling another adult how patient and understanding she has been. Your child loves to hear you bragging about her.

Make sure teachers and other adults in your child's life know the impact of the health situation.

> *A neighbor I didn't know very well spent a lot of time talking to my son about what it was like to have a little sister who was sick all the time. It turns out she had first-hand experience when she was his age. She really did a great job of letting him vent. I don't think he wanted to talk to me about this because he didn't want to upset me.*

If a sibling is having a lot of trouble, look for a counselor who has experience helping children deal with an illness in the family.

Child-Care

Whether you are going out to dinner with your spouse or returning to employment, leaving your infant or child with reflux in the care of others may seem like the last thing you want to do. You may have feelings of protectiveness. You may think she will only take a bottle if you feed her or that a childcare provider won't know what to do when she starts shrieking. In other words, no one can replace you in the child-care department.

You may feel pressure from others to let go, have some fun or go out on a date with your spouse. But you are just not ready - yet. Be sure to verbalize your fears and concerns to others. Make it clear to your spouse that you would LOVE to carve out some couples time like in your "before reflux" days. Your spouse needs to know that you are not choosing one over the other. It is just that you have to feel comfortable allowing someone else to care for the baby.

Letting Go

It may take some extra planning for you to be able to let go. You may need to start slowly by allowing a family member to care for the baby while you are in another part of the house. Dad, grandma or a family friend may be the obvious choice because they are invested in the baby and know you and your family best.

The first time somebody else cares for the baby, it may be best to have them watch your techniques so you can show them your caretaking routine that resulted from your many hours of trial and error. Try to give them a little room to develop their own techniques, but they should accept your instructions and follow your wishes.

Eventually, you may feel comfortable going out of the house for an hour or two. Remember, things may go better or worse than expected. Try to be patient and realize that everyone is doing the best they can.

> *My husband forced me to get out of the house by arranging a few hours at a salon. I felt like a queen for the day. I spent the morning getting my hair and nails done and then went out to lunch with a friend. I called about a million times to see how they were doing. My husband told me that everything was under control. It has made such a big difference in my life to go out after being isolated so long.*

Making the Decision to go back to Work

The reality is that many mothers delay their return to work until the reflux is under control. It is often necessary to extend leave or take leave without pay.

> *I stay home but not because we were able to afford it. We make it happen. I do some part-time work in the evenings when my husband is home. We always get what we need each month, but it isn't easy. In fact, some months we take turns with what bill we will pay.*

It's a juggling act when we don't have enough money, but leaving my daughter would have been much harder.

When the time comes to return to work, you may feel guilty that you won't be able to take care of your baby during the day. It may seem that you spent so much time caring for your baby during the worse of the reflux that there was little time to really enjoy her. Now that she is feeling better, you want to be there for every smile and playful moment. Now someone else will be there for those important milestones.

When it came time for me to go back to work, I was frantic with worry that he would be miserable with the sitter. I delayed and delayed until it was clear that I would lose my dream job if I didn't go back at least part-time. I interviewed sitters and was delighted to find two who both had lots of experience with reflux in their own kids. One had fewer kids in her care we hired her. The other had her hands full, but offered to be the back-up person if the regular sitter got overwhelmed. I was so touched!

Finding a Good Match

You will need to spend some time looking at all of the options and deciding what type of care situation you prefer and then selecting a provider. Some parents chose in-home care so that their baby gets one-to-one care. In this type of situation, you have more control over how your child is cared for and the schedule.

I have taught a class on reflux to home daycare providers several times. I'm always impressed with their great instincts about how to care for these babies. Even the providers who didn't know the term 'reflux' could still tell me exactly what spitty babies need.

A group child-care situation allows your child to be around other children, which may help a picky eater experience a positive feeding environment. Don't hesitate to clearly state the needs of your child and ask the doctor for a note if needed. The good thing is that there are multiple caregivers so nobody gets too burned out caring for your fussy little one. And with more caregivers, you increase the chance that somebody at the center will have first-hand knowledge of reflux.

Every time he vomited, the daycare center called and told me to come and get him. The daycare rule says that a child who has vomited needs to be separated from the other children and picked up right away. I talked to the director and explained that he had reflux but she still had to follow the procedures. After this happened a few times, I had the doctor write a note explaining that the vomiting was from reflux.

◆

My story: My daughter needed a pacifier because of her reflux so the doctor wrote a prescription. The daycare provider was concerned that the other kids would be jealous so we sewed the pacifier to a stuffed monkey and said it was his. My daughter was allowed to "borrow" it from the monkey only at naptime when the other kids weren't watching.

You need to find a child-care provider who you feel comfortable with. By communicating effectively and working together as a team, your child will thrive.

You may have a lot of worries about going back to work and finding day care. You may worry that a caretaker won't be as patient about the crying and vomiting as you. You know how frustrated you get, what about a child-care provider? Will she take care of her like I do and hold her after meals like I instructed her to? Be sure to discuss all your worries with your new team member.

Care and Keeping of Your Child-Care Provider

Once you have found a wonderful child-care provider, it is important to support her and let her know how important she is to you and your family. Let her share her feelings and concerns with you. It is important to keep the lines of communication open so you can both ask questions and resolve problems effectively.

She may have concerns and questions about the reflux too. Be sure to communicate information from the doctor. You may even want to invite her to a doctor's appointment so she can hear the recommendations directly and report to the doctor what she is seeing from her point of view.

It is vitally important to provide extra support and encouragement to a child-care provider who must care for a high-need baby or child all day. You know how exhausted you feel after a full day of holding and comforting. Your child-care provider must feel the same way. Verbalize these feelings and watch for signs that she is feeling stressed.

If your daycare provider is watching your child in your home, she may be isolated from other adults. In a daycare center, the child-care providers can give each other a break to eat lunch or care for a less needy child. Perhaps you or your spouse can come home from work occasionally so your child-care provider gets a moment to regroup. Perhaps a friend or relative can come during a busy time of day such as mealtime or late afternoon when your baby is most fussy or needy. On particularly bad days, you might want to have a special reward - buy pizza for your daycare provider's family.

Communication

You may want to develop a system of communication such as a notebook or chart to write down observations. Your child-care provider needs to know about a rough, sleepless night just as much as you need to know about vomiting episodes during the day. Find a quick, easy system such as a checklist.

It may be helpful to write down instructions for each task such as feeding, medication, tummy time, etc. Be sure to develop a plan for emergencies before one occurs.

Shaken Baby Syndrome Worries

In rare cases, a child-care provider has shaken a baby and caused injury. This is a terrifying thought for all parents. You already know that taking care of your high-need baby can be exhausting and may cause feelings of anger. You need to talk with your child-care provider about how to handle a situation where she gets to the end of her rope. Should she call you? Should she bring the baby to a neighbor? Should she put the baby in her crib and close the door and then call you? Make it clear that you would be grateful to receive a call for assistance and you would admire her for knowing when she has gotten to the point where she can't go on. Remind her periodically about your concern for her and the plan for this type of situation.

Notes:

13 SLEEP OR LACK THEREOF

Daytime parenting is an exercise in patience and stamina, even on a good day. When your child has acid reflux episodes at night, you may have your endurance tested further.

This chapter will cover typical sleep patterns seen in infants and toddlers with reflux. There are many hints on getting your baby to sleep so you can get some rest too. The chapter on positioning and home care has specific information on sleep positions and devices such as wedges to elevate the bed for sleeping.

Why is Sleep so Difficult?

During the day, your baby is probably upright most of the time. The esophagus is in a vertical or upright position. She has a greater chance of keeping food in the stomach and may experience less pain from reflux when upright.

At night, a baby sleeping on a flat surface doesn't have gravity to help keep the food in the stomach since the esophagus is horizontal. There is a better chance that the stomach contents will escape from the stomach and enter the esophagus. We all know what happens from there. The acid irritates the esophagus or causes choking and begins the night waking cycle once again. Now you understand why it is possible to have a relatively happy baby by day and a screaming baby at night.

At the same time that gravity and positioning are, allowing more reflux episodes, the LES or lower esophageal sphincter may also fall asleep on the job. During sleep, children with reflux also experience a decrease in swallowing and saliva, which help to wash down the reflux during the day.

Just when you thought there could not be any more bad news, other potential sleep grabbers are added to the mix. A typical respiratory illness, teething or ear pain/pressure can aggravate reflux and contribute to night waking. Other babies wake up at night due to discomfort from food allergies, enlarged tonsils and constipation. Breathing issues such as sleep apnea, asthma and choking on secretions can jolt gerdlings and their parents from a sound sleep.

Sleep Affects Behavior and Health

When children don't sleep well, it can lead to attention, learning and memory problems as well as aggression and tantrums. Chronic sleep problems may leave children more susceptible to infection and illness.

Even adults say sleep and reflux don't mix!

A recent Gallup study indicated that a high percentage of adults with acid reflux report night waking, night pain and difficulty getting uninterrupted sleep. Poor sleep due to acid reflux is the most difficult quality of life issues they face. The interrupted sleep affects their ability to concentrate during the day and work effectively. No wonder our babies are crying out in the night!

Typical Sleep Patterns for Babies and Toddlers with Reflux

While we know there is a range of "normal" sleep patterns for infants and children, it is likely that reflux has prevented any type of normal sleep pattern or routine in your household. Since you have already read all of the baby books, we will spare you all of the details about what is "average" and "normal."

A few babies with reflux sleep well. But the vast majority have serious problems getting to sleep or staying asleep.

My baby won't sleep. A twenty-minute nap every few hours is not enough.

◆

The moment her little head hits the crib, she starts wailing.

◆

I haven't had a full night sleep in over three months. It feels like years.

◆

My baby wakes up at night in pain. She is not just jerking my chain.

◆

My twins still wake up every few hours - never at the same time, of course.

Poor Sleep, 24/7: This baby is a poor napper, poor sleeper and seems to sleep less than other babies of similar age and weight. She may take short catnaps during the day or not sleep at all. She may only sleep on your shoulder or in a sling or carrier. She doesn't sleep more than a few hours at night without waking up.

Awake All Day, Sleeps All Night: She tends to take short naps during the day or stay awake all day, even in early infancy. However, she may sleep for a long stretch of the night.

He was so exhausted from being awake all day that he somehow managed to stay asleep all night. I know most parents of babies with reflux have babies that don't sleep well at all. I think my guy is just exhausted.

Painful Wake up Call: This baby wakes from a deep sleep in intense pain. She is difficult to console.

It is amazing. She will be sleeping completely soundly when I check on her, but minutes later, she will wake up shrieking at the top of her lungs. She is clearly exhausted and angry that the pain woke her and it is very hard to get her settled down.

Light Sleeper: The light sleeper, wakes with the least sound. You tiptoe around the house while she is napping and lunge for the phone on the first ring. She may also cry out in her sleep, move all over the bed or kick and thrash.

She just cannot find a comfortable sleep position. I hear her tossing and turning, kicking the rail of the crib and whimpering in her sleep. Eventually the pain breaks through and she wakes up.

Wants to Eat All Night: This baby wakes frequently and seems to want to eat, even after the newborn period and when weight is within a normal range. Your baby may want to drink something to wash the acid out of her esophagus. Or she may not be getting enough calories during the day.

Our 9 month old usually wakes several times at night to eat and eats full, big bottles - getting much of his needed calories at night when he is more relaxed and able to eat. (Unlike day feedings which rarely exceed 3 oz).

Difficulty Falling Asleep: She falls asleep easily in your arms but wakes up the moment you place her in her crib. The pain of reflux prevents her from being able to fall asleep unless you are comforting her and holding her upright.

I walk with him until my arms are aching.

Coughing, Choking and Other Scary Sounds: Coughing and choking can interrupt her sleep. Parents often check on this little one because she makes so much noise.

I heard the gulping and the grunting on the baby monitor and knew that I would be out of my warm bed any minute now.

Sleeps almost all the time: Over the years, we have heard about a few babies with reflux who sleep more than twenty hours per day. This seems to be their way of avoiding the pain they feel. It might seem like a blessing, but a baby who sleeps this much won't have time to practice skills like eating and playing.

How Bad is It?

After such a full day of caretaking, you really deserve a good night's sleep. Your aching body is crying for rest and your brain cannot process another shred of information.

Your whole being needs to rest. You don't even need a bed. You are so tired you could sleep standing up. Even the sofa or rug looks like a fine place to sleep.

Just as you are placing your head on your pillow, there is a familiar sound. Your baby is crying, no shrieking...again. Because you are a parent, you are instantly awake. The sound of your baby calling you is a sound that pierces your body and wakes your brain from a deep sleep. You are the parent of a baby with reflux so your baby wakes often and you find yourself on the night shift.

As a parent, you don't need a sleep deprivation study to tell you what you already know. Not getting enough sleep leaves you feeling drained and tired all day. You may also feel like your brain doesn't work and you can't think clearly, even for the simplest task. Adults who do not get enough sleep are at risk for illness, accidents and poor job performance.

Many parents also report feeling irritable, angry or depressed. Sleep deprivation may change the way you react to problems large and small. You may have less patience and get upset faster. A little problem may seem huge when you are exhausted. During the day, the first person you see (i.e. spouse, doctor) may get a big share of misplaced anger just from being in the wrong place at the wrong time. At night, you may feel exhausted and angry at your baby for waking you up again.

Some babies seem to choke, cough and hold their breath. Of course, you are going to be on high alert day and night. How could you NOT worry? What is any doctor or grandparent going to tell you that will make you feel less worried? Your parenting instincts are telling you something is wrong and you have to stay nearby night and day.

So how are your supposed to sleep? Your brain tells you to stay awake but your body is craving sleep. You train your brain and your body to "hear" in your sleep and wake up at the slightest change of her breathing.

Most parenting books tell you to sleep when your baby sleeps. This parenting advice works just grand if you only have one baby, if you have live in staff including a housekeeper, nanny and cook and you don't have to work outside of the home. Otherwise, you may find yourself taking a shower, paying the bills or throwing in a load of laundry the moment you get the baby peeled off your shoulder. You are positively joyful about being able to move faster and bend over without whacking her in the head as you get some basic chores done.

It can make a tremendous difference if you take at least an occasional nap. Another way to get some sleep is to take a break from the night shift by having your spouse handle the night waking too.

> *Once the baby went to sleep in the afternoon, I would curl up on the couch and take a 30-minute nap. My preschoolers knew that mommy was not to be disturbed and they were not to leave the room unless the house was burning down. They usually watched an educational video or played quietly on the floor. When the video was over, they knew it was safe to wake me!*

> *There were so many nights that I went to bed just as soon as the kids were tucked in. Some nights, I got my best sleep between 8pm and midnight before the night waking would start.*

Tips for Getting a Baby with Reflux to Sleep

If your baby is in pain, nothing you do is likely to make her sleep well. The best advice to help your baby sleep is to work with your doctor to control the symptoms that cause night waking.

When the reflux has been under control for at least several weeks, you can begin teaching your baby to go to sleep and stay asleep.

Positioning

The chapter on home care and positioning provides many options for finding a comfortable sleep position and elevating the bed if the doctor has recommended it.

Co-Sleeping

In many cultures, it is accepted practice for an infant or toddler to sleep with her parents. In this country, it is expected that babies will sleep in their own crib in a separate room. Some parents believe that sharing the bed makes it easier to nurse and care for a baby who wakes up frequently. Parents also report that they feel closer to their baby and more in touch with their needs.

I tried everything and found that co-sleeping in a bed was the best way to get the most sleep possible. I will be honest, I co-slept with my daughter until age three and still do sometimes. I refused to let her cry-it-out as long as I knew she suffered from reflux. Let me tell you she is the best at going to sleep now at three years old.

When we put the baby in our bed, none of us got any sleep. We compromised by putting a large mattress on the floor in his room and one of us would go sleep with him when he needed it.

Decrease or Eliminate Night Feeding

Many babies with reflux sleep better when their stomach is empty. Your doctor may recommend decreasing or eliminating night feeding after six months unless weight gain is an issue and 24 hour a day feedings are medically necessary. If your baby absolutely needs a drink at night, see if you can wean her to water only. Keep an eye on weight gain if you and your doctor decide to try this. Hopefully, she will take more calories during the day when she is more comfortable.

I was still doing night feedings at seven months to get the calories in her. My GI doc promised me if I stopped night feedings she would make up for it during the day, and she has. She has slow motility issues and during the night, motility is always slower in everyone so really night feeding was bad for her. It was a difficult decision because she really, really needed the calories, but I saw her sleep so soundly after I cut the night feedings.

Sleep Environment

Make it clear that night is for sleeping, not playing. The room should remain dark and quiet.

Most babies go through a stage where they wake at night wanting to play. You can discourage this by acting like the most boring person in the world. If she sees that you don't want to play and will barely cuddle, she won't try as hard to stay awake.

Reflux made my daughter very clingy. She never wanted to be out of my sight. Because of the reflux, she was afraid of her crib. After the reflux was gone, she still wanted to sleep with me but she was SO restless and I would end up with bruises from her little toes digging into me at night or I would wake at 3 am to find her pulling my

*eyelids open to see if I wanted to play. Our solution was for me to
sleep on the floor next to her crib for a few weeks until she realized
the crib was safe. She could watch me sleep but not wake me up.
When she was older, we let her come in our room and sit in the big
chair and watch us sleep. We increased her independence without
ever letting her feel abandoned.*

If you have to change diapers at night, do it quietly and keep the lights
low. If the sheet is covered with vomit, place a thick towel over it rather
than changing the whole bed. Tuck the edges in securely so she can't
pull it over her face.

Take a Nap

One thing that parents have noticed is that reflux gets worse when the
baby is overly tired. Your baby may act like she doesn't want to sleep
during the day, but her body might need more rest to function better. Try
hard to create a relaxing, boring time during the day. If her only options
are sleeping or staring at the walls, she might sleep.

Earlier Bedtime

Sometimes, the only way to get more sleep is to go to bed earlier. As a
society, we are used to running till we drop and then expecting to fall
asleep instantly. But many babies and adults sleep better if they go to
bed when they are tired, but not exhausted.

Why Letting Her Cry it Out May Not Work

If your baby woke up every two hours due to pain from an ear infection,
would family and friends advise you to let her cry-it-out at night? If
your adult friend came to work yawning after being up all night with
acid reflux, would you tell him to just deal with the pain at night and go
back to sleep? Most likely the answer would be no in both cases. So
why do family, friends and even physicians tell you that it is ok to let
your little one cry it out when she wakes up at night due to reflux?

It is likely that reflux is causing the night waking so letting her cry-it-out
just won't work. In time, the reflux will get better and she will learn to
sleep.

*When she was about 15 months old, I read a book about teaching
your baby to sleep. I tried the techniques a few nights. I would go
into her room and place her back down in the crib and rub her back*

before leaving the room. Of course, she continued to cry. It was just awful for both of us. I finally stopped when I walked into her room the next day and saw the big puddle of spit-up on her sheets and on the floor. She was so upset that she had vomited.

Calming Baby by the Book

There are several excellent books that teach parents simple but effective techniques to calm their baby and help them to sleep. It is likely that there will be some excellent ideas for a refluxer too. Try not to blame yourself or the book if the advice isn't totally effective for you. Remember, your baby has a medical condition that may make calming and comforting extra challenging. There are many excellent books on the market, but a few books recommend techniques that are just too harsh for a baby who has sleep issues because of pain.

We started trying Dr. Karp's Happiest Baby method when our son was going on 3 months old. The shushing and jiggling worked well to calm him. The swaddling worked sometimes to calm him but if I left him swaddled too long he would get very angry all over again. So once he was calm for about 1/2 hour I would unwrap him. I told the pediatrician about the book, and if I ever knew another woman who was going through what we have with the reflux/colic I would get her a copy. I think the method would have worked even better if we had learned about it earlier and swaddled him earlier. If you've only seen Dr. Karp on TV, you should know there is soooo much more in the book and video than what is shown on TV.

It is certainly a good idea to establish healthy sleep habits from an early age. However, you need to be careful about your expectations when you child may be experiencing pain. I read every book at the library and studied each theory...and she still could not sleep at night. It wasn't until she had adequate pain management that she was able to sleep well. I must say that reading the books and understanding the mechanics of helping a child to sleep helped her develop good habits. When she was able to sleep at night, she did it without training or dramatics. I helped her associate going to sleep with a special object - blanket, stuffed animal, etc. so that I was not the only "special object" to help her go off to sleep. I gradually shortened the time we spent together rocking in the rocking chair over a period of weeks until we were down to a minute or two. If she woke up at night, I kept the lights off and tried not to get her out of

her crib. Again, it could take months just to achieve this step. There were constant set backs because she had a lot of illnesses so we would just go back to square one and start over again. My daughter now has no trouble falling asleep by herself and sleeps well. All of the "bad habits" I had - nursing her to sleep, rocking her to sleep, bringing her into my bed, holding her when she was crying and frantic at night, etc. didn't damage her too much! I don't have any regrets!

Take it Slowly

There may be setbacks and problems along the way. It may seem that the reflux is getting better and then a new tooth erupts or your little one catches the cough that is going around. Remember, it took a while to get into this situation; it will take some time and patience to get out.

My doctor said that it can take many months of being out of pain till her sleep problems will be fully gone. He says if the problem took three months to develop, you can expect it will take about six months to fully solve. It is already much better but we have a ways to go.

◆

During the year my daughter did not sleep through the night, I thought that I was losing my mind. I am usually very organized and I found myself misplacing the phone bill or driving the wrong way to the food store. When I talked to people, I couldn't remember words or names of people. It was very demoralizing. People make jokes about "new mother haze" but I had it for much longer! I am happy to report that it is a survivable condition and my daughter did eventually learn to sleep all night. Surprisingly, most of my brainpower has returned too!!

◆

Posted: Stop worrying about what everybody else thinks about how to raise YOUR daughter. First, follow the instincts you have as a mother. If you think your daughter is more comforted sleeping with you, then sleep with her. If sleep problems arise later, then you can deal with them later. Don't worry about later...you will deal with whatever happens later, later! Focus on right now and how you can make right now easier. Sleep problems can happen regardless of how they are put to sleep now or where they go to sleep now. What is more important is that you and her are comfortable now. If you are bothered by opposing opinions (like I am from close family and friends) then don't share it with anyone. It really isn't anyone else's business but your own. They don't live with her, you do. It isn't their child, it is yours. Do what you and your husband think is best.

Notes:

Section 2

Advanced

Concepts

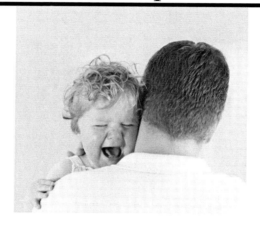

This section of the book is for families of children with more severe reflux, older children and children with multiple medical problems. The earlier chapters of the book cover the basics. Please read them first.

14 TESTING

Testing is not generally needed to diagnose reflux, but babies and children who have confusing symptoms or do not respond to treatment may benefit from further testing.

While the Testing chapter is full of detailed descriptions of the common tests used to diagnose reflux disease, your child may not need any of them. It may be tempting to read about the other tests and suggest to the doctor that a particular test is needed. If your child has already been diagnosed with reflux and you end up persuading the doctor to perform the test, don't be disappointed when you get the results - you might just end up with a test report that states, "The patient has reflux!"

Questions to Ask the Doctor

The news that your baby needs a test may stir up a great deal of anxiety and stress. No one likes to subject their baby or child to medical procedures, sedation and X-rays. It is important to understand fully what will happen during the test and what information the test will yield. By asking questions and letting the doctor know your concerns, you can work together to make the best decision for your child and you will feel more confident about doing the test.

The doctor's office will provide specific information such as location of the test, arrival time along with fasting and medication instructions. Make sure you understand the doctor's orders and ask questions well before the day of the test. There may be different restrictions depending on the age of your baby, whether you are breastfeeding, etc.

Questions to Help Make the Decision:

What is the goal of testing? What are you trying to learn?
How is the test performed?
Can you treat her without doing a test?
What are the risks involved? Sedation, exposure to X-rays, discomfort, fear, risk of infection?
Is there another test that will answer our questions better?

Logistical Questions

Can I be there during the test? Or until she is asleep?
Will it be painful or uncomfortable? How can we remedy this?
What type of sedation is best for my child?
Where will the test be done? In the office? The hospital?
What time should we arrive?
How long will we be there?
Are there eating restrictions before the test?
Should she have her medication the day of the test?
What should I bring?
Is she allowed to have a toy or a blanket?
Is there a TV or other bedside entertainment?
Should she wear/not wear certain clothes?
When will we know the results?

There may be other practicalities to attend to as well. Certainly many insurance plans require pre-authorization and a written referral. If the test requires fasting or traveling a distance to a far away location, you might need to make additional arrangements. Perhaps you will want to pack a small bag with extra clothes, food and other necessities in case there is a delay or schedule change. It is often helpful to bring a family member or friend to help you on the day of the test and offer moral support. It is unlikely siblings will be allowed in the testing area.

Preparing Your Child

Keep in mind that each test is different and each child reacts differently. There are may different hints for preparing your child for each test in this chapter. Hopefully, some will work for your child.

Here are some common concerns and solutions for helping you and your child cope with testing.

Managing Anxiety

A baby or toddler may be completely unaware of the testing. What your little one will be most afraid of is being separated from you and being in a room full of strangers. It might help to bring some familiar items from home such as a favorite blanket or teddy as well as a cool new toy to offer diversion.

Often the parents are much more traumatized by testing than the children are. For the most part the children are asleep and don't remember a thing. Sometimes parents are anxious about being separated from their baby. Be sure to tell the staff your concerns.

> *I kept saying, "I don't want to be there for the actual procedure but I want to be with my toddler until she is asleep and then see her as soon as she wakes up." The staff didn't exactly understand that. They kicked me out of the room before she was very sleepy and she got upset when she saw me leave. When they finally allowed me in the recovery room, she had been awake for a while and she was howling. Next time, I will be more insistent. Just a few extra minutes on each end would have made a huge difference.*

If your baby or toddler has been a frequent flier at the doctor's office, she may develop a fear of the whole medical environment. Some toddlers and young children begin to whimper as soon as the car pulls up to the doctors office and it is all downhill from there.

It might help to give a toddler the opportunity to play with a doctor kit. The local toy store should have a child-sized version of medical tools for a young child. Let her pretend to give you a shot or fix your boo- boo with bandages and kisses.

Some doctor's offices and hospitals provide special play therapists to help a child get ready for a medical procedure. Ask your doctor about this well ahead of time.

> *I was so grateful for the "Play Lady" as my daughter called her. The Play Lady helped us put a gown on a doll, put on a bandage and in-sert an IV. My daughter clutched that doll during the whole day in the hospital and proudly showed it to her friends in preschool. It*

made a world of difference in her attitude to talk about the procedure ahead of time.

Bribery can be an amazing tool to help your child build good memories after a traumatic event. If it helps, buy your child a toy on the way home from the really traumatic doctor's visits.

Managing Pain

It is very helpful to alert the doctor ahead of time if you know your child has a very low pain threshold or extreme anxiety about medical procedures. The doctor may be able to prescribe medication or even a special lollipop (Fentanyl) that has relaxing medication before the tests.

We are so lucky to have a doctor who makes full use of all the pain control and relaxation techniques. Before a test, I can give my son a "chill pill" before we even leave the house. And we have a tube of numbing medicine that completely takes away the pain from the IV. After he is a bit relaxed, I spread the medicine on his arm where the doctor showed me and cover it with a bit of plastic wrap. It takes a while to get numb, but by the time we get to the hospital, he can't feel a thing.

There are a number of products designed to ease the pain. Most take over 30 minutes to work so you will need to plan ahead.

A key part of managing pain is managing fear of pain. Once your child becomes afraid of pain, the pain will be harder to control. If you see that your child is becoming afraid because she knows that something painful is coming, you need to work with the medical team to get her to trust you again. This means not inflicting more pain.

Hospitals are required to use pain scales, but there are many studies that show that pain in children is very under-treated.

Explaining the Test to Your Child

An older child may want more of an explanation of the procedure but remember that you don't need to be too graphic. Use words they can understand and explain things from their point of view. In addition, offer reassurance that you will be there as much as possible.

Before the endoscopy, I told my toddler, "After you get on your special pajamas, you and Teddy will take a ride on the magic bed and take a little nap. I will be waiting for you right here. Tell Teddy to stay awake and tell us all about it. Afterwards, you can have a grape ice pop and watch the dragon DVD."

◆

We found a great book on endoscopies that is available from the Prevakids web site. It is called My Endoscopy Story By Jack.

Common Tests

Testing can be used to prove the presence of reflux, measure damage, monitor progress, guide treatment or identify other medical issues that affect the success of the treatment.

Upper GI Series

The Test

An Upper Gastrointestinal Series or Upper GI (UGI) is the most common test administered to children with symptoms of reflux. An Upper GI is not used to "prove" reflux, it is used to "rule out" other conditions.

The test provides a view of the digestive tract (mouth to stomach) to detect a structural problem. An upper GI is used to rule out a structural problem or birth defect of the stomach. An Upper GI can give a rough idea if the stomach is emptying too slowly, but a milk scan is a more sensitive test for this.

Even if the child vomits during an Upper GI, it doesn't necessarily mean that the child has reflux. The child might simply have been upset and vomited. Reflux is only diagnosed based on a pattern of excessive backwashing of acid or when the backwash is causing problems and this test is too short to show a pattern of reflux events.

A mother called me right after her baby had an Upper GI Series in a state of confusion. She reported that the radiologist said there was no evidence of reflux. How can that be? My baby clearly has all of the symptoms. I explained that the Upper GI showed that her baby didn't have a structural problem (REALLY good news) and her baby somehow managed NOT to reflux during the test. I said, "So what

*happened after the test was over?" She said, "Well, he vomited all
over the car on the ride home." I said, "That was the reflux part."*

How the Test is Done

Soft tissues such as the stomach and intestines do not show up well on
an X-ray. An Upper GI consists of having the child drink a chalky liquid
and taking an X-ray of the stomach. The chalky substance has barium in
it which makes the outline of the stomach easier to visualize. A normal
X-ray is designed to show hard substances like bone. Upper GI testing is
usually very quick and you can expect to take your child home right
away.

What You Need to Know:

The test will be performed on an empty stomach so you will not be able
to feed your baby for several hours before the test. You may be asked to
bring a bottle of her favorite formula, milk or expressed breast milk. The
technicians will put barium in the bottle and ask you to feed your baby.
If you are pregnant, you may need to let somebody else feed your baby
and stay for the X-ray because the test involves exposure to a small
amount of radiation. It might be a good idea to bring your own bottle or
sippy cup to increase the chances your baby or child will drink the barium.

The barium powder tastes like chalk, but most young babies don't object
much if they are hungry enough. Older children may not like the chalky
feel of the barium "milk shake" and it can cause nausea.

Wrestling your child and forcing food into her mouth may be counter-
productive if she is already afraid of eating. It may actually make the
situation worse if the gag reflex is stimulated and the child vomits the
barium before the X-ray can be taken. The results of this struggle can be
seen clearly on many X-rays - there appears to be more barium outside
of the child than inside! It might be necessary to place a small tube into
the child's stomach and pour the barium through the tube.

Your baby may be placed on an elevated surface or wrapped on a special board or papoose to keep her from moving around too much. She
might be very unhappy with this aspect of the test. The good news is,
parents are usually allowed to stay during the test and the test only takes
a few minutes.

Being in the car- seat contraption to hold him still seemed to bother him much more than drinking the barium and formula mixture.

Some parents wear a hospital gown so they are protected from possible vomiting during and after the test. You may want to bring a change of clothes for both of you just in case. Some children experience constipation and white, chalky stools after a test. When the test is over, your baby can resume eating and drinking. Bring a bucket for the car ride home, just in case. Mostly, you will both need a good, long nap.

They put a tube down his nose and throat to put the barium into his stomach. Then he was strapped to a board (while they took the X-rays) and he screamed. At least I was able to hold his hand. It broke my heart but I can assure you that two minutes after, he'd forgotten about it already. I bought him a new stuffed toy at the hospital gift shop - to make myself feel better.

Variation - Modified Barium Swallow Study

A swallow study is similar to an Upper GI Series. A swallow study is used to assess the mechanics of swallowing and evaluate a swallowing disorder, also known as dysphagia.

Your baby needs to drink the barium and milk mixture during the X-ray. A speech pathologist who specializes in swallowing may be in the room during the test. The swallow is recorded on video and played at slow speed to see how your baby swallows.

The test is also used to see if food is entering the airway during a swallow or if the food is getting into the stomach properly but being refluxed up and getting into the lungs later.

PH Probe Test

A pH probe is an acid monitoring device that measures the acid level in the esophagus and gives an indication of reflux severity. The test also measures the frequency and duration of reflux episodes.

The probe records data and provides the doctor with detailed information about the reflux events. The data is complex and often entered into a computer scoring program to help the doctor grade the severity. For instance, if your child has one very long acid event, it may be more important than a lot of short events.

A pH probe test is considered to be an excellent test to confirm reflux, however, a few children with significant reflux have had "unremarkable" or "negative" pH probe tests on occasion.

> I couldn't believe it when the doctor called and told me that the pH probe results were largely "unremarkable." How could that be? Overall, his reflux is just as bad as it has always been. Now what do we do? I'm so confused. Is he just very sensitive to acid or did he have a good day?

Some doctors perform a probe while a child is on reflux medication to check the effectiveness of the treatment. Most often, the medicines are stopped a few days before the test because the goal is to see if the child has reflux without medication.

How the Test is Done

A thin, flexible tube is threaded up through the nose and down into the esophagus. The tube looks like aquarium tubing. It is as thin and almost as flexible as cooked spaghetti. There is a small sensor at the end. The tubing is attached to a small box that records acid events.

In general, the test takes approximately 24 hours and many hospitals require the children to stay overnight. Older children may be able to leave the hospital after the tube is inserted and go home for the duration of the test.

The probe is attached to a small box with a shoulder strap or backpack. A digital readout allows you to look at the current level of acid and get an instant reading on whether certain activities provoke reflux events. You will be asked to keep a diary to record what your child is doing during the day. This helps the doctor spot activities that provoke reflux - lying down, eating, crying or jumping on the couch. Some parents find it overwhelming to juggle all of these duties for 24 hours.

What You Need to Know

Your baby or child will not be allowed to eat for a few hours prior to the test. Sometimes the doctor will perform an endoscopy first and then place the pH probe while your baby is still asleep. If not, the probe will be placed while your child is awake.

The placement of the tube may be the hardest part of all. While it isn't really painful to place the tube, it will be uncomfortable and scary to many children. Putting a tube in your nose just doesn't feel good. Some doctors provide a spray to numb the nose before getting started.

It is important for your little one to be very still for the few seconds it takes to place the probe to avoid injury. Infants and toddlers may be swaddled or placed on a special board to keep them from moving. A nurse may be there to keep the child still and assist the doctor with the insertion. Parents may be allowed to stay for the tube placement and can provide a soothing voice and some distraction. An X-ray is often needed to check the placement of the probe before your baby can resume eating.

> My toddler just had a pH probe study. The worst part was inserting the probe into his nose. I wasn't in the room but I could hear him crying from down the hall. I know he had to be held down and that sure did make him mad.

Your child will probably be quite annoyed about being restrained and having the tube placed. She will also dislike the tape on her cheek to keep the tube from moving around and the irritation to her throat from the tube. She may cough and clear her throat in an attempt to adjust to the tube. In general, be prepared for a grumpy, unhappy child for the first few hours. Be sure to bring several new toys to provide a distraction.

Keeping the probe in place can be as much of a challenge as placing it in the first place. Babies and toddlers will not be able to understand that they can't yank the tubing out of their nose. Mittens are routinely placed over babies' hands to prevent them from pulling the tube out. Most toddlers will need to wear inflatable arm splints, elbow restraints or some other method of immobilizing the elbows so she can't reach her face. Nurses call these No-Nos. Ask if the hospital provides them or if you need to buy/make your own. Brand names to look for are Heelbo, Posey, Imak, SnuggleWraps and AliMed.

Older children may keep their hands away from the tubing if they are provided distractions such as videos and books.

The nurse brought mittens to put on my toddlers hands to keep her from tugging at the probe. This was clearly not enough, so the we had to use arm splints that prevented her from touching her face.

If your child will be hospitalized for the pH probe, you will need to pack some essential items such as clothes, toys and food. Your child may be able to wear regular clothes and pajamas so check with the hospital before hand so you can be prepared. It might help to bring some favorite foods and eating utensils such as bottles, sippy cups and familiar bibs so you can replicate diet and eating habits as much as possible. You want to have your child eat, sleep and play as normally as possible to obtain an accurate test.

At first, your child might not want to eat because it feels strange to swallow with the tube in place. She might be groggy if she was sedated.

He vomited the first feeding after the insertion, but after a few hours, the probe didn't seem to bother him too much.

A picky eater may reject everything on the hospital menu so ask the nurse for help with selecting foods. There may be a small kitchen on each floor with juice, crackers and cereal. Most hospitals will allow you to bring food and heat it in their microwave or have it delivered from a nearby restaurant. Ask ahead.

My 5 year old was starving and eager to eat. She brightened when the tray was delivered and quickly opened the lid covering the plate. We both gasped at the same time: my world famous picky eater with severe acid reflux was served a southwestern omelet complete with salsa, onions and green pepper! Luckily, the nurse came to our rescue and was able to get a replacement meal quickly. Afterwards, I was able to laugh about it, but at the time, it was not a bit funny!

You and your child should be able to visit the playroom and perhaps even go to other parts of the hospital such as the gift shop or cafeteria. While you probably don't want to encourage gymnastics, you should certainly be as active as possible.

I found it a challenge to chase around after him in the hospital room with the pH monitor attached. The nurse told us there was a wagon we could use to take a little walk. My son was thrilled to pack up his train book and his blanket to take a "train ride." It was a relief to keep him busy and distracted, even for a few minutes.

Variation - Dual Channel pH Probe

Many hospitals are purchasing probes with two sensors. These can be particularly useful if the child has confusing symptoms. One probe can be placed in the lower esophagus and one in the stomach if reflux is suspected. Sometimes the two probes are positioned so one is in the lower esophagus and one in the upper esophagus. This helps to detect whether the acid is getting all the way up into the mouth or airway.

A pH probe may not detect when alkaline pancreatic enzymes backwash from the small intestine into the stomach and then into the esophagus. This alkaline reflux may not show up on a standard, single-probe device because the alkaline enzymes combine with the acid in the stomach and register a neutral pH level. Unfortunately, the pancreatic enzymes are still capable of causing severe damage

Alkaline reflux should be considered a possibility if the child has symptoms of reflux but a relatively normal pH study. Reviewing the computer data of the pH probe to search for evidence of alkaline events may be productive or the child may need to have a dual probe pH, Multi Channel Intraluminal Impedance or a Bilitec test. (below)

Variation - Multi-Channel Intraluminal Impedance

The Multi-Channel Intraluminal Impedance Test (MII) is a newer, more sophisticated version of a pH probe, which can sense acid and nonacid events. Unfortunately, it is not widely available at this time.

While a traditional pH probe may have two sensors, the MMI has additional sensors along the length of the tubing. These special sensors can detect the difference between food that is being swallowed (going down) and food that is being refluxed (going up). It is also possible to detect liquid in the esophagus and episodes of reflux that are not acidic. Nonacid, non-alkaline episodes that are not picked up by a pH sensor are recorded on the impedance sensors. It is believed that non-acid, non-alkaline reflux can still cause problems such as choking for some children.

Variation - Pharyngeal Airway pH Monitor

A new device is available that monitors acid vapors at the back of the mouth where the airway and mouth join. It is mostly available for researchers, but a few hospitals have the Restech Dx-pH Measurement

System. The probe goes up the nose and the tip sits just at the back of the throat.

Variation – Bravo pH test

The Bravo Probe is a wireless pH monitor. The probe is about the size of a gel capsule. It is attached to the inside of the esophagus and transmits data for 48 hours to a recorder the size of a pager. It is less embarrassing and patients report it is more comfortable because there is no tubing touching the back of the throat or sticking out the nose.

Variation – Bilitec

The Bilitec measures the presence of both acid and bilirubin that has backwashed from the small intestine through the stomach and into the esophagus. Certain foods interfere with the testing.

Upper Endoscopy

An endoscope (en-DOSS-kuh-PEE) is a device (flexible fiber optic tube) attached to a camera that allows a doctor to see into the body. It allows the doctor to view the walls of the esophagus, stomach and the upper part of the intestine.

How the Test is Done

An endoscopy is often done in a procedure room at the hospital with general anesthesia. Some hospitals prefer to use sedation or "twilight sleep" rather than full anesthesia. There are benefits and drawbacks to each and you should discuss this with the doctor well ahead of time.

During the test, the end of the scope is carefully inserted into the mouth and down the esophagus. The doctor will advance the scope slowly and watch on a video monitor. If a problem area is seen, a camera or a video tape can be used to record the image.

An endoscope lets the gastroenterologist observe visible damage to the esophagus such as swelling, scaring or ulcerations. It can also allow for observation of the lower esophageal sphincter opening and closing. The scope can be used to view problems in the stomach such as ulcers or gastritis. An endoscopy can also show if there are any rare birth defects of the esophagus such as a spot where the esophagus has fused to the airway.

What You Need to Know

The hardest part of an endoscopy for your child is the test preparation and sedation. Procedures for preparing a child for sedation vary from hospital to hospital. A child may receive medication to relax them and make them drowsy. The doctor may use a mask to provide a small amount of medication to make the child fall asleep for a few minutes. The masks often smell like fruit or bubble gum to make it more appealing to a child. Some doctors wait until the child is asleep to start an IV while others insert an IV when the child is awake.

After the test it will be necessary stay for a period of observation. Your child will be offered a drink and you will probably go home with instructions to resume eating and activity as tolerated.

Biopsy

Some types of damage may not be visible to the naked eye. Biopsies (small samples of tissue) will be taken during the endoscopy to check for microscopic damage, signs of allergies and the bacteria that cause ulcers.

Tissue samples taken during a biopsy are checked with a microscope for changes that can occur as a result of chronic damage. When the cells are exposed to acid for many years, they can start to change.

One common change is the presence of white blood cells called eosinophils. These cells belong in the blood stream, not in the digestive system. The significance of eosinophils in the digestive system is not entirely clear. A small number of eosinophils in the esophagus probably means that acid exposure has occurred and the eosinophils are present as a part of the healing process. However, large numbers of eosinophils may mean your child has Eosinophilic Esophagitis, a condition that is related to allergies and appears to be increasing dramatically in children. Eosinophilic Esophagitis and reflux look nearly identical but have different treatments so it is important to check for this disease.

Biopsies are one way of testing for the presence of helicobacter pylori, the bacteria implicated in ulcers. The significance of h.pylori is the subject of much debate. If a biopsy shows your child has h.pylori, please consult up-to-date medical literature.

Small bowel biopsies may be taken if there is any reason to suspect that your child has celiac disease, an intolerance to gluten. The symptoms of celiac disease are very vague in children and doctors are beginning to test for it in children who have digestive issues or are small for their age. Treatment consists of avoiding wheat, barley, rye and oats. These grains contain gluten, which eventually damages the lining of the intestines.

Food Allergy Testing

There are several clues that food sensitivities may be involved in your child's reflux: a history of skin rashes such as hives or eczema, breathing problems such as asthma or wheezing, constipation, chronic diarrhea, blood in the stools or a family history of allergies.

Our understanding of allergies and food reactions has changed dramatically in the past few years and is still changing rapidly. New research shows there may be several different types of food reactions. Food allergies may produce obvious, fast symptoms or symptoms that come on many hours after eating the food and can be very hard to spot. There also seems to be a category of food reactions that don't show up on tests because they are not true allergies.

The most common food allergies in children are: milk, eggs, peanuts, tree nuts, fish, seafood, soy and wheat.

Many parents explore food allergies but only a few have dramatic success stories where avoiding a few foods completely cures the reflux. There are many other stories where eliminating foods helps but does not completely eliminate the reflux.

> *Everybody in our family has allergies including some very strange ones like ice and vibrations. I was really hoping we would find an allergic basis for my daughter's reflux. But we had no luck at all.*

Allergy testing is a bit controversial because there are many tests and they are not all accurate in all circumstances. A test may show a "false negative" which is a situation where a food does cause trouble but the test fails to show there is a problem. "False positives" are also common – the test shows an allergy and you avoid a food that really isn't causing problems. It appears that false results are more common in the youngest patients. While there is some controversy about the accuracy of allergy testing in infants and young children, it is indicated in some situations.

It is important to find an allergist who likes to work with food allergies and who has experience working with infants and young children. There are societies of allergists and several patient support groups that may be able to help you learn more about current allergy theories.

Testing Methods

Skin tests are the most common test for food allergies. A drop of food is applied to the child's back and then scratched lightly into the skin. After a period of time, the skin is checked for redness or hives (raised, itchy spots).

> We figured that the skin testing would show our baby was allergic to a few foods. We were surprised to find she is allergic to several more than we thought.

Patch tests are a new type of skin testing that may demonstrate "slow" allergies. It involves saturating a tiny band-aid with a food and sticking it on the patient for several days.

Blood tests called RAST or ELISA may be an option to test for food allergies. Some patients prefer a single blood test over a skin test involving multiple pricks/scratches. They may not be as accurate for every type of allergy.

Another strategy to "test" for food allergies is to try a short (7-14 day) elimination diet. Under the supervision of a doctor, a strict diet is adhered to. After a week or more, one food is added back to the diet each day. The theory is if the symptoms go away when a food or food group is taken out of the diet, the food was the cause of the symptoms. Likewise, if you add the food back to the diet and symptoms return, it confirms the role of the food in causing symptoms. Elimination diets are quite difficult and there are entire books to guide you.

> My son's reflux is absolutely allergy driven. When I was nursing, I eliminated milk, eggs, soy, nuts, chocolate, beef and several other foods. It was a huge amount of work and the pediatrician didn't think it was worth it. As far as we are concerned, it is worth the expense and hassle. We found one allergy book that had information on re-

*flux – Is This Your Child? By Doris Rapp, MD. It has great instruc-
tions for doing your own detective work.*

Scintigraphy

Scintigraphy (sin TIG ruh fee) or a scintiscan is often referred to as a
milk scan or delayed emptying test. It is used to track the progress of
food as it moves out of the stomach (gastric emptying) and through the
digestive system and rule out delayed emptying. A doctor may also use
scintigraphy to detect aspiration of food into the lungs. The test can detect reflux episodes, but it too expensive and too much of a hassle to use
it just to confirm reflux.

What You Need to Know

The test is performed in the nuclear medicine department or radiology
department. The radiologist will place a small amount of radioactive
material in a drink you provide (milk, formula or breast milk).Your
child needs to drink at least 2-4 ounces for the test to be reliable. Older
children may be given food instead of a liquid. Usually scrambled eggs.

Find out ahead of time if the doctor has a preference for adding the
powder to a liquid, a thick liquid or a solid. You and your doctor need to
decide which would give the most useful information. Ask if you
should bring the food from home.

Some parents are concerned about the idea of their baby or child ingesting the radioactive material for the test. The material is excreted when
the child has a bowel movement and does not stay in the body perma-
nently.

To conduct the test, it is necessary for the child to lie still for about an
hour. An infant or toddler may need to be swaddled or strapped onto a
papoose board to keep them from moving. A blanket or pacifier may be
helpful for an infant. An older child may be able to cooperate and lie
still on the table for the duration of the test when provided ear phones
for music or other distraction. Some testing facilities have TV's and
videos for the children to watch. It is always a good idea to bring your
own bag of tricks - a book, music and earphones.

After the first hour of testing, your child can get up for an hour or so and play. Unfortunately, the test has two parts so she will need to go back on the table again. Luckily, the second half of the test is a lot shorter.

Your child may think this test is a very bad idea and may cry the whole time. You can ask for medication to help her relax. If you are lucky, your little one will fall into an exhausted sleep at some point.

Less Common Tests

These tests are often used to rule out medical conditions that have some of the same symptoms as reflux.

Esophageal Manometry

Manometry is a test to rule out swallowing disorders or an overly tight Lower Esophageal Sphincter (achalasia). A small flexible tube is placed in the esophagus (or intestines) and measures the strength of the muscle contractions that move food through the digestive system. The child may be asked to drink or swallow during the test.

Lactose and Sugar Intolerance Testing

An inability to digest sugars such as lactose, fructose, mannitol, sorbitol may cause symptoms that look like reflux. Lactose intolerance is relatively easy to treat and it is easily mistaken for reflux in some children.

Symptoms of lactose intolerance include burping, gassiness, bloating, diarrhea and constipation. It is caused by the inability to digest lactose, a digestive sugar that naturally occurs in milk. There are many lactose free foods and formulas as well as over-the-counter medications, which help break down lactose.

Your doctor may suggest an elimination diet or a breath hydrogen test to rule out a lactose or other sugar intolerance.

Malabsorption Testing

There are three basic reasons for poor weight gain – too few calories going in, too many calories being lost due to vomiting, or the body isn't using the calories and other nutrients at a typical rate. Children with very poor weight gain may need to have testing to be sure they are absorbing and using nutrients properly. This can include testing for fats, vitamins or minerals.

Gluten Intolerance Testing

Celiac Disease (CD) is an inability to digest gluten found in wheat, barley, rye and oats. Patients with CD who consume gluten for years eventually develop damage to the lining of the intestines and this can lead to severe malnutrition. Early symptoms of CD look like reflux. Biopsies can detect later stages of celiac. Antibody and genetic testing are also available. Please consult current medical literature for the pros and cons of the various tests.

Electrogastrogram / EGG

Electrogastrogram (also called electrogastrography) is a way of measuring the electrical impulses that control the grinding and pushing muscles of the stomach. It is very similar to an EEG (electroencephalogram) which measures brain waves. It is used to rule poor contraction of the stomach (gastroparesis) which has symptoms similar to reflux.

Sleep Study

During a sleep study, the child is hooked up to machines that monitor breathing, brain waves and a pH probe to learn whether reflux is causing sleep disturbances.

Small Bowel Transit Testing

If slow intestinal motility is suspected of causing the reflux, a test can be done that determines the amount of time it takes a meal to move through the intestine. There are several tests. One of the common ones involves having the child swallows markers (tiny plastic beads) that can later be tracked on an X-ray. Different shaped markers are swallowed several hours apart.

Sweat Test

A Sweat Test is used to rule out Cystic Fibrosis (CF). Cystic Fibrosis is a rare condition characterized by severe breathing and digestive problems causing poor weight gain. Hundreds of PAGER kids have had this test over the years and not one test has ever come back positive.

When the pulmonologist said she needed a test for Cystic Fibrosis, I was shocked. The doctor saw the panicked look on my face and

*quickly added that it was highly unlikely she had CF. The doctor ex-
plained that CF is extremely rare but early detection is very important. Of course, the test came out negative. I think they call it a
"sweat test" because it makes the parents so worried that they start
to perspire!*

Notes:

15 REFLUX IN OLDER CHILDREN

Many people are familiar with infant reflux and adult reflux, but few people realize how many older children have reflux. It is estimated that reflux affects several million children in the United States. Unfortunately, many older children are under-diagnosed and under-treated for their symptoms because reflux symptoms are often mistaken for stress, a poor diet or behavior problems.

Treating and diagnosing older children is usually the same as treating and diagnosing an infant. You will want to read some of the earlier chapters for detailed information about these topics. This chapter gives you information that is not covered in the earlier chapters such as dental care, going to school and participating in sports.

Note: If you are a parent of a baby with reflux, it may be discouraging to read this section. We have provided this information for those who need it. Remember, most babies outgrow reflux and you will probably never need the information in this chapter.

You might be reading this chapter because your older child has just been diagnosed with reflux. Perhaps your child started having symptoms out of the blue. For most families, this is just a continuation of reflux that started in infancy. First, you had the screaming spitter followed by the world's pickiest eater at age two. Just when you thought you couldn't stand another moment, you found yourself explaining to the teacher about your child's digestive system.

We thought our daughter's reflux was long gone, but when she was three, she started to tell us about icky wet burps after meals.

You may be wondering if the reflux will ever go away and if your life will get back to normal. The good news is that over time, most children and their families learn to manage reflux and get control over the symptoms. They do everything that other kids do, they just do it carefully.

Symptoms in Older Children

Older children tend to have slightly different symptoms than babies. Instead of spitting up or vomiting, they might have stomach pain or a sensation of food coming up the esophagus. A child may have one symptom or many. The symptoms may change over time as the child grows and matures. Please read the basic symptoms chapter first.

Pain: Abdominal pain above the belly button, chest pain, heartburn, burning in throat, pain with swallowing, bloating/fullness. Rare: pain that radiates to the top of the shoulder joint or the shoulder blade.

Food Coming Up: Silent reflux, wet/sour burps and belches, wet hiccups, vomit in throat, sensation of food coming up into the throat and even the nose. Rare: nausea, vomiting, feeling of food being stuck in the esophagus.

Picky Eating: Extremely picky about food, avoids specific foods or food groups, certain textures are rejected, reports that certain foods cause pain/burning during or after eating.

Weight Issues: Poor or slow weight gain is very common. Some children are overweight due to constant eating and drinking to push the acid back down. Rare: weight loss.

Sleep: Poor sleep, night waking, pain and heartburn when lying down, coughing. Rare: sleeping excessively to avoid pain, choking.

Behavior: Anxiety, depression, poor attention or behavioral problems.

Respiratory: Chronic sore throat, frequent colds, chronic or recurring sinus infections, bronchitis, pneumonia, wheezing, asthma, night cough, throat clearing, hoarse/deep voice, hiccups, ear infections or ear pain. Rare: laryngospasm (severe type of choking), apnea and sleep disorders.

Dental: Bad breath, excessive saliva, large cavities, "moon cavities" which are shallow and affect the points of molars. Rare: tooth enamel erosion affecting the sides of the teeth.

Esophagus: Esophagitis. Rare: esophageal ulcers, strictures. Extremely Rare: Barrett's Esophagus (pre-cancerous condition).

Headaches: In one study of children with GERD, frequent headaches were reported by many of the participants. GERD is one possible trigger for migraines.

Diagnosis

It is a bit easier to diagnose reflux in an older child than an infant because they can report their symptoms and concerns to the doctor. Even a very young child should be encouraged to tell the doctor where it hurts and what foods bother her.

Sometimes parents and children have special code names for reflux. One little girl would tell her mom she had "yucky stuff" in her mouth. Another child would tell her mother, "I have a crumb in my throat." Constant communication helps you to track the symptoms and document the frequency of the problem since many children don't have a good concept of time.

> *My son is a bit shy and doesn't like to tell me about his symptoms. He thinks discussing reflux is as gross as talking about pooping and peeing. We use a chart where he can mark his symptoms.*

The doctor will ask you many questions, look at rate of growth and conduct a physical exam before making a diagnosis of reflux.

Is It All in Her Head?

Your child's doctor has to explore all reasons for stomach pain and there are many children who react to stress by getting stomachaches.
Your doctor may wonder if your child's frequent stomachaches and visits to the school nurse are related to stress or school anxiety. He may refer your child to a counselor or psychiatrist to see if stress is causing her symptoms.

Even though reflux is not caused by stress, it can be aggravated by stress. When a child is in pain and feels like the adults around her don't understand, this can be an enormous burden. A counselor can help your child verbalize her feelings and develop coping strategies.

> *My daughter was furious when the doctor sent her to a counselor. She thought this meant the doctor didn't believe her. She may have been correct, but the counseling was a great idea. Before long, the two of them were getting along wonderfully and now my daughter has a great outlook on her illness. The counselor says she was suffering from Post Traumatic Stress Disorder from all the medical treatment when she was younger.*

> *The doctor thought my daughter's stress level was causing her reflux and suggested counseling. After several sessions, the counselor wrote a letter to the doctor stating that my kid is very well adjusted considering her pain level and made it clear that the stress came after the disease.*

Treatment

Older children benefit from many of the same treatments as young children such as lifestyle modifications, medication and a special diet. The ideas in this section go beyond the baby advice that is in the first chapters of the book. See the various treatment chapters for a full description of the treatments available.

Sleep Positioning

If your child wakes up at night or seems tired after a full night in bed, it might help to elevate the head of the bed. You may have to try several strategies to get your child comfortably elevated.

Some children do fine with an extra pillow or two. A wedge pillow is preferable because it elevates the whole torso and avoids bending the stomach.

Try using bed blocks under the head of the bed. They are available at most bedding stores. The blocks may be stacked to gain extra height.

If you raise the head of the bed too much, your child will start sliding down. You can try to put wedges or regular pillows under her thighs and calves to elevate her knees - look at the way a hospital bed raises at the knees to prevent the patient from slipping. Flannel sheets or pajama bottoms with feet may help prevent slipping.

Some children feel comfortable sleeping in a recliner chair.

Several of the manufacturers who make reflux devices for babies custom make them for older children (and adults) as well.

There is an inflatable wedge for travel.

Many adults with reflux sleep in a recliner chair. There are many child size recliner chairs on the market. You can put fitted sheets on them to keep them clean

You may have to do something extra to secure the sheets to the bed when the mattress is elevated. Look for sheet suspenders at bedding stores or ask a friend who sews to alter the sheets so they go further around the back of the mattress.

Loose Clothing

Your older child may want to wear the latest fashion trends. Hopefully, the "style of the week" will include wearing loosely fitting clothes around the waist. Tights, tight fitting jeans and pants may put more pressure on the stomach causing reflux episodes.

Medication

You will want to read the chapter on giving medications to learn the basic tricks for flavoring and compounding for babies. These additional tips may be helpful for older children.

Older children may have strong opinions and attitudes about medication. Some children like a particular flavor of liquid medication and others like a pill to swallow quickly without any taste. Let your doctor know what works best so they can prescribe a liquid, dissolving tablet or pill depending on your child's preferences.

Give your child a simple explanation about why she needs the medication. If your child seems reluctant to take medication, try to figure out why. Is it giving her a headache or is she objecting to the taste? Some children need some kind of incentive like a happy-face chart or other reward system.

An older child may want to assist in measuring and preparing medication as a way to feel in control. In most cases, it is a good idea to foster independence and good self-care habits. Just remind her that a parent must always be present during medication time. She might get confused between an over-the-counter antacid (fruit flavored, chewy) and candy.

> We didn't keep the antacids locked up because we didn't feel like they were real medicine. My neighbor found my daughter giving them to her kids. Now we keep them locked and we had a long talk.

Avoid Tobacco and Alcohol

When she was little, you had complete control over her environment. Now that your child spends some time away from your house, be sure to tell her that it is important to avoid tobacco because it aggravates reflux. This includes second-hand smoke. Have her practice what she will say or do when other people want to smoke around her.

> When people smoke around our son, it really bothers his stomach and lungs. He tells people that the doctor says he can't be exposed to smoke. He can't bring himself to tell them to stop, but at least he makes it clear that he can't be nearby. All the men in our family started smoking young. I'm proud that he isn't taking up my former bad habit.

Alcoholic beverages and alcohol in liquid medicines makes the LES relax and aggravates reflux. At least one of the reflux medications (ranitidine) should never be taken with alcohol.

Going to the Dentist

Some children with reflux have a higher rate of tooth enamel erosion due to acid reflux. More research is needed to determine how common this problem is and how to prevent it. Meanwhile, children with reflux need to be monitored closely by the dentist from the moment the first tooth comes in. You will receive instruction on careful brushing and other treatments to protect the teeth. It is a good idea to encourage your child to rinse out her mouth with water following a reflux episode.

> My 4-year-old gerdling has one or more cavities at each check up even though I am so careful to help her brush her teeth and the dentist seals every molar as soon as it comes in. My nonrefluxer is 11 years old and still has not had one cavity.

Your refluxer may complain that the toothpaste tastes bad or causes reflux. You may want to experiment with other brands or try toothpaste for sensitive teeth. Brushing with water is not as effective as using toothpaste, but it is better than nothing.

A child with oral motor sensitivity or a strong gag reflex may resist tooth brushing completely. You may need to monitor tooth brushing and work with the dentist or a speech therapist for further assistance. Electric toothbrushes can help.

> *The pediatric dentist always has a big selection of flavors of toothpaste and fluoride treatments. While the dental hygienist proudly recites the list, my refluxer has a pained look on her face and I know she is thinking...Banana? Yuck. Orange Cream? Not in a million years. Grape? Double Yuck. Do I have to choose? They all sound bad to me! Why isn't there an unflavored?*

Behavior and Emotional Issues

Your refluxer may need a different kind of parenting to deal with the special circumstances of having a chronic health condition. Sometimes you have to bend the rules a little if your child isn't feeling well. If it seems like the "well" periods are so short that there is little time when things are normal, you may need to be exceptionally creative in your approach.

> *She was pushing my buttons all day with her misbehavior. That night, she didn't eat her dinner and then she vomited. Her reflux was acting up again. No wonder she was so hard to live with! I felt bad that I had lost my patience with her and put her in time out.*

> *When I think my child is misbehaving, I ask myself how I would be acting if I had a migraine. I know I'm very short tempered. I don't let her misbehave, but I do correct her more gently or just take her home. Later, we discuss how her reflux made her grouchy.*

> *My husband thought that we babied our son too much when he was sick. He said we were creating a "mama's boy." Yes, we treated him differently than our other kids, but he needed the special care. In the end, he turned out to be well adjusted.*

◆

My mother is amazing. She really remembers what it is like to be a kid. My reflux prevented me from participating in about half the things I wanted to do at school and with my friends. My mom knows that an important part of being a teen is having friends and learning to have balance in your life. Even if I missed some school because of my reflux, she made sure I didn't miss all the social activities, too.

A child in chronic pain may exhibit a wide range of behaviors from withdrawn to overly active, upset or agitated.

When she would come back from a birthday party, she would collapse in a heap of tears. I would hold her on my lap and the truth would come out. It wasn't friends being mean, it was the cake that made her feel bad.

One important lesson that babies learn is that adults can fix whatever is wrong. The minute she cries, you come running and fix the problem. If your baby is in pain all the time, she may not learn the type of trust that most babies have for their parents. She needs to feel that you are trying your hardest to fix the pain.

If your child is chronically ill, she may have developed some fears and phobias about doctors and medical care. Crying, resisting treatment and temper tantrums may be her way of expressing fear and distress. You may need to work with the medical staff to help her verbalize her concerns and work through behavioral issues. If the problems persist, seek counseling for her.

My story: Katie was afraid of anything having to do with doctors. Glasses, white coats, stethoscopes and even Band Aids. One year Santa brought several boxes of colorful band-aids. My daughter had fun being the doctor rather than the victim. Every person and doll in the neighborhood was covered with Band Aids by the end of the day.

All children like rules and routines. Having a schedule and a predictable sequence to the day makes everyone feel more in control. Often, school provides this type of secure, predictable routine as well. If your child is missing school often due to illness, she may feel out of step with her friends. She may need more routine at home to make up for missing her routines at school.

If chronic pain is affecting her school performance or behavior at home, talk to the doctor about treatment to manage the pain better.

Going to School

It may be hard to let your little one go to preschool. You both have been through so much together and it may seem a little scary for both of you. You may have concerns about all of the "what ifs." What if she needs me? What if she doesn't feel well? What if she cries for me? What if everybody thinks she is spoiled?

Your child will look to you for cues about how to behave. It is important for you to give her permission and confidence as she steps forward toward independence. Take your time and do things in small steps when necessary. Plan for the what ifs. Let the adults know where to find you in an emergency and about the special care she needs (diet, medication, extra snacks).

Help your child think of an easy way to explain reflux when the need arises. Some children explain that they have acid reflux while others simply say, "My doctor said I have to eat a snack" or "My reflux makes me burp really loud."

You are still the most precious person in the world to her, perhaps in a deeper sense since you have been on such an important journey together. She will always remember the special closeness and return to you after her adventure into the big world.

Your child may need to eat a special diet or eat frequent small meals to manage her reflux while at school, just like at home. It may be necessary to meet with the school nurse and teacher to develop a plan for the classroom. School schedules and policies may get in the way of good eating to manage reflux.

It isn't always easy to convince the school staff about the importance of following a treatment plan. Your child may look as healthy as the other kids in the class so it may not seem that medical treatment is needed.

My daughter had a hard time eating lunch with her class since it was the last lunch period of the day. If she didn't eat a snack in the late morning when the hunger pains started, she would get a stomach-ache. By the time her lunch period would come, she was so hungry that she inhaled her food and ingested a lot of air. This caused bloating and pain that lasted the rest of the afternoon. We had to make sure she had a snack or the day was a total loss.

Sometimes a school nurse or teacher will believe that a stomachache is a sign that a child is trying to avoid school or has an emotional problem. It may be necessary for the doctor to write a letter to the school describing the situation and the treatment that is needed during the school day. The law is clear that the doctor's recommendations must be followed at school.

The doctor wrote a note on his prescription pad for the school. The note stated that my daughter was to have drinks and snacks at her desk throughout the day.

Some children are not at all bothered by the disease and all the special attention. They are proud of their burps and think it is funny to start a burping contest with the whole class. But other children find all of this unwanted attention can cause your child a great deal of embarrassment. She may feel strange that she is the only one allowed to have food at her desk.

My son was really self-conscious about eating his snack at his desk. Day after day, he told me that he wasn't really hungry and didn't need it. I started giving him snacks that he could eat without being noticed - forget noisy wrappers or crunchy food. He kept a baggie of breakfast cereal or crackers on his lap and took out one piece at a time when no one was looking.

Be sure to talk to your child about school and develop a plan together. Check in periodically and make sure everything is going smoothly. It is also important to check in with the school staff and thank them for help-ing your child.

A whole booklet on going to school with reflux is available from PAGER Association and www.reflux.org.

Sports

Some children find that certain sports such as wrestling and weight lifting put too much pressure on abdominal muscles, leading to increased reflux episodes. Sports like swimming and gymnastics can provoke reflux because of the horizontal or upside down body positions.

With the proper medical treatment and diet, your child should be able to participate in most sports. You and your child may need to experiment with diet and see if light eating before exercise can help. Well-timed medication such as before a sporting event also helps a lot. Consult your child's physician or a sports medicine specialist for advice. Doctors who work with athletes are often very familiar with reflux treatments and tricks.

You Know You Have a Child with Reflux When...

Friends, relatives and strangers tell you, "She looks so healthy." "She doesn't look sick." You just nod and smile.

The pediatrician says, "All babies" cry, vomit and wake up at night. But your baby is inconsolable for hours at a time, vomits 30+ times a day and does not sleep more than an hour.

Your husband, friends, neighbors and grandparents refuse to be left alone with your high-need baby. Those who do come to help never return after one day at your house.

You have to buy a new car seat every few months because the old one reeks of vomit and special formula.

You struggle to stay awake while driving home from the food store at 2 o'clock in the afternoon. You are sure a policeman will pull you over for weaving and revoke your license on the spot.

You have not had a full night of sleep in (fill in the blank) years. You know the sleep deprivation studies are correct.

Your baby vomits so much she has ruined a chair and the new carpeting. You both run out of clean clothes by 10am each day.

You seek support/info on the internet. Most of the time, you don't get a chance to log on until 11:30pm. Sometimes you hold the baby over your shoulder with one hand and hunt and peck with the other hand.

You finally get out to enjoy a leisurely lunch with the other reflux moms. Half way through the meal, you realize that the other patrons in the restaurant are listening in horror to your conversation containing graphic descriptions of body fluids - color, quantity, frequency, amount of blood, which end, etc. You think this is funny.

After caring for your inconsolable baby 24/7, you know why babies are shaken or worse by their parents.

Instead of joining the moms and tots playgroup or the PTA, you joined PAGER, Mothers of Asthmatics and the Food and Allergy Network.

You have taken multi-tasking to a new and dangerous level.

You and your child have watched far too many videos due to frequent, prolonged illnesses. You quote Disney movies at cocktail parties and hum the theme song while during laundry. You have watched Toy Story 68 times.

You always have a contingency plan.

Instead of reading, "What to Expect in the First Year," your parent bookshelf contains: Physician Desk Reference, a good medical dictionary and the Merck Manual (physicians edition, not the home edition).

You keep meticulous records. You are sure your child's food intake record contains clues for an effective weight loss plan. You plan to publish it, make a lot of money and appear on Oprah.

The baby book is full of cute mementoes - hospital bracelets, picture with Santa on Christmas morning in the children's ward, discharge orders from surgery.

Your pediatric gastroenterologist carries your child's records with him at all times. He tells you his vacation/leave plans before the front office staff.

Your child's medical records at the pediatricians office is so large, it has to be divided into Part I and Part II by the time your child is 7 years old.

You've fired doctors, had heated debates with others and stood your ground when the doctor dismissed your concerns or tried to discharge you too early. You know the saying is true, when you have a sick kid, "Don't mess with the mama lion."

You are positively ecstatic when both the specialists can see your child on the same day at the children's hospital an hour away. Imagine what you will do with all of that free time!

To visit grandma, Disneyworld or go camping for the weekend, you pack a large tote bag full of medicine, syringes, tubing, stethoscope, starter supply of antibiotics, AC adapter for the durable medical equipment, a case of special formula, a feeding pump and a nebulizer. You worry that you have left something vital behind.

The FAA issues a travel alert warning of delays when your family plans to travel by air due to the excess baggage and security screening involved.

You don't have to "panic buy" before a snowstorm or hurricane. You learned a long time ago to be prepared for sudden illness, a trip to the hospital and being homebound for days or weeks at a time.

The drugstore pharmacist at the mega-food store knows you by name despite the fact that they fill thousands of prescriptions per month. On average, for every $100 you spend on groceries, you spent $50.00 on medication and formula.

You pack an overnight bag before a sick visit to the pediatrician. Often, you need it and wish you had packed more chocolate bars.

Your little gerdling has 50+ doctor/clinic appointments and 75+ prescription refills per year.

An overnight stay at the hospital feels like a mini vacation after managing your child's illness at home. Reality sets in when you are discharged and resume your 24-hour duties as pediatrician, nurse, gastroenterologist, nutritionist, pharmacist, respiratory therapist, social worker, case manager, housekeeper, laundry aide, video changer on top of your other household/family duties. You envy the nurses who get to go home after a 12-hour shift.

You know you will survive this because of your friends, family and organizations such as PAGER Association are there to support and guide you.

You and your child have developed a special bond. You wonder if you would cherish your child as much if her chronic condition hadn't forced you to spend so much time together.

You wonder if you would have learned to live in the present and appreciate the little things if your child didn't have a chronic illness. You didn't think your life would be like this. You have no regrets and wouldn't change one little thing.

Notes:

16 FEEDING YOUR OLDER CHILD

If your toddler is happily eating stage-three food from a jar and grabbing your bagel while she sits on your lap, there is no need to read this section. If she doesn't seem thrilled with sitting in a high chair and eating from a spoon or she cries during a meal, read on.

If your school age child eats pizza and soda or at least two foods from each of the major food groups, don't worry too much. But if she needs rocks in her pockets on a windy day to keep from blowing away, read on.

You should read this chapter if:

Your child's food list contains only a handful of items such as apple juice, crackers and chicken nuggets

Your child strictly adheres to the "White Diet" or "Prison diet" of rice, pasta, bread, mashed potatoes, chicken and saltines

You keep a food diary

You show signs of "waitress syndrome" - you cook special meals for your child and spend hours in the kitchen

You follow your child around the house with a bowl of food or a sippy cup and attempt to feed a sip here, a bite there

You call Grandma to celebrate when your child eats 3 bites of food in a meal

You feel angry and defeated about feeding your child

You can't even tell when your child is hungry - her signals are very confusing

It seems like you work much too hard to get your child to eat compared to other parents

You have read every book on picky eating and none of it seems to apply to your child

This has all been going on far too long to just be a phase

The Careful Eater

A child with reflux often eats a small variety of foods and eats a small quantity of food. In addition, she may limit her intake to mushy foods. She may be a grazer, eating a bit here, a bit there all day long. She is often a carbo junkie-craving starchy foods such as potatoes, crackers and bread. She may avoid many foods that other kids will eat.

Children with reflux often become very careful eaters because they have found, through trial and error, that certain foods, literally, leave a bad taste in their mouth.

Foods can trigger pain, burping, bloating, stomach or chest pain or a burning sensation in the throat. Older children report that they can taste the food they ate an hour ago. Bending over or engaging in vigorous activity after a meal can trigger symptoms. Wouldn't you be a picky eater if you tasted vomit and acid in your mouth after every meal?!

> *I never let people call my child with reflux a picky eater. Just as someone who is allergic to peanuts is careful, even vigilant, about avoiding peanuts at all costs, a child with reflux is careful about avoiding foods that trigger a reflux episode*

> *One of the hardest things about reflux is that others don't understand that your child doesn't want to eat and the stress that causes. If I had a dollar for everybody who suggested I try chocolate because all kids like it, I would be rich. Most gerdlings HATE chocolate!*

Feeding a preschooler or older child with reflux can be very time consuming and difficult. It is easy to blame yourself for feeding problems. But remember, it takes two to tango. You and your child need to interact and work together to make feeding successful. It is your job to provide healthy foods at appropriate intervals and it is the job of your child to eat familiar foods, try new foods occasionally and acquire new feeding skills. If she doesn't, you need to find out why rather than blame your-self.

It may feel like you caused your child to become a picky eater. Perhaps you developed "waitress syndrome" out of desperation to get your child to eat anything. Maybe you bought pretty plates and fancy straws to encourage your child to have a good attitude about eating. The bottom line is your child has a medical condition that makes feeding difficult for everyone. But remember this: your picky eater will most likely eat you out of house and home by adolescence – as long as you don't push them too hard before their stomachs are ready.

> It seemed like she was a picky eater forever - chicken, potatoes and rice. Over and over...But over time she started to try a lick here, a lick there. Now she eats just like any other child. It took her a long time to trust foods.

Feeding Aversion

A child may be labeled as having a feeding aversion or feeding disorder if careful eating escalates to an extreme level. A child with a food aver-sion may eat a small number of foods and have very strong reactions when you attempt to give her any other foods. She might throw a major tantrum if you deny her the foods she prefers. You don't dare put a new food on her plate since it is likely to cause loud complaining!

If you can count the number of foods your child eats on one hand, whole food groups are missing from your child's diet or your child seems afraid to eat, it is time to start addressing this issue.

> His reflux seems to be under control with medication. We are now dealing with the ramifications of reflux in the most extreme way - re-fusal to eat. Our son is wonderful except when it comes to food. He used to live on a nutritional drink, water and the occasional bite of a cracker. Now, we have a terrific feeding specialist who has lots of experience and he is starting to have a better attitude about food af-ter just a few sessions. The first step is more flavorful crackers, and now you can see he is intrigued.

◆

> We really thought the reflux was gone and he hadn't been on reflux medicine for months. The whole family was convinced that he just didn't want to eat anything other than macaroni and cheese. Even I

thought he was just being picky. We talked to the doctor and decided to try medication for two weeks before going to a feeding therapist. We were all surprised that he started eating better after a week. The reflux wasn't gone, but he had never complained of pain, he just didn't want to eat.

When a child is admitted to a feeding clinic for a feeding disorder, the first thing they do is rule out a medical reason for the poor eating. Usually, acid reflux plays a big role in causing the feeding problem.

Parents complain that they are often blamed by family, friends and physicians for creating a picky eater. A few years ago, we asked the director of a large feeding clinic how many of the kids referred to the clinic have acid reflux. He stated, "If they don't come in with a diagnosis of acid reflux, they leave with a diagnosis of reflux because it was missed all along."

It may be necessary to consult with a feeding specialist or a feeding team to manage the discomfort from eating and decrease behavioral patterns that developed because of the pain of eating.

Tips for Feeding Your Toddler and Older Child

It is important to manage reflux symptoms and pain through diet and medication. A child will have a great deal of anxiety about eating if each bite leads to pain and discomfort. The other tips and tricks just won't work very well if your child is in pain.

Remember that children on acid reducing medications will be more susceptible to food poisoning. They don't have acid in their stomach that can kill bacteria in food. Be sure foods are properly refrigerated and throw leftovers away after three days. There is also a theoretical concern that genetically modified (Bt) corn could be bad for patients with reduced stomach acid.

Timing Meals

Small frequent meals are often recommended to ensure that the stomach isn't too stretched from a large intake of food. Your child may benefit from a small meal every few hours during the day.

> *Instead of saying, "Snack Time" (which implies cookies and sugary juice), I named the snacks for the foods we would eat. In the morning, we always had our "Fruit Snack" and in the afternoon, we always had our "Yogurt Snack." After they had consumed the main snack food, they could nibble on other foods such as crackers.*

Some children experience pain if they are too hungry so they nibble and graze all day so a bit of food is churning in their stomach all day. Dr. Sears tells his patients to eat half as much but twice as often. Chewing thoroughly can make a big difference in how long a food takes to digest.

Your child may have an "eating window," often from mid morning until late afternoon where eating is less painful and the most calories are consumed. If your child is attending school during this important eating opportunity, it is vital to arrange with the school for healthy eating.

> *My daughter could not face food until 11am but then she was ready for a full meal. Her eating pattern really messed up my routine because I was not used to cooking at noon and again for an evening meal. I soon found some short cuts and was turning out a hot lunch without too much added time in the kitchen. When she started school, she was allowed to take a protein shake in an insulated mug and slurp it all morning.*

Quiet Play Following a Meal

While is fine for most children, children with reflux may develop significant pain from engaging in physical activities right after a meal. It is best to encourage quiet play after meals. Try story time, puzzles or an art activity rather than vigorous play. Activities like jumping on the couch and chasing the dog may be best on an empty stomach. Older children often have recess or free play just after lunch, which isn't the best time.

Most children also benefit from scheduling meals at least an hour before bedtime so their stomachs are empty when they lay down.

Reflux Diet

Parents always want to know if there is a special diet to manage reflux. Unfortunately, there is not a recommended diet or cookbook.

Many children with reflux naturally find that a high carbohydrate diet reduces discomfort. This is affectionately called the White Diet or Prison Diet by many. Children find that white foods such as crackers, pasta, cereal, potatoes and rice are easily digested. These foods are out of the stomach quickly and converted to energy. While many children consume adequate calories on the White Diet, there is some concern that the diet lacks key nutrients because meat, dairy, fruits and vegetables are largely absent from this diet.

The general rule is that children with reflux should eat the foods they can tolerate. Each child reacts to different foods. Don't restrict your child from all the foods listed below – just the ones that bother her.

Many refluxers find that eating spicy foods can trigger reflux symptoms. Sometimes bland food is not appealing and you may find you can entice your girdling with foods that have some zip that doesn't come from hot spices. Try herbs or salt. Even a bit of sugar might convince her to eat something she might not normally like.

Acidic foods such as oranges, lemons, tomatoes or vinegar can trigger reflux symptoms. Some parents find that using Prelief Sprinkes (acid reducer for food) can cut the acidity of foods like orange juice and spaghetti sauce so they can be enjoyed.

Foods that cause gas and belching can induce reflux. Beans, broccoli cabbage, onions, cucumbers and some other foods may cause gas and bloating. Beans can be soaked several times to cut the amount of burping and gas they cause. Drain off the soaking water. You can also cook them with epizote (herb) or Beano.

High fat foods may trigger symptoms because fats digest very slowly. Babies and toddlers need some fat in their diets so consult your physician before putting your young child on a low-fat diet. Foods such as donuts and creamy sauces are full of fat.

Other children find that it makes a difference whether the food is raw, cooked, frozen or canned. Sometimes this is because cooking changes the acidity and other times it seems to be the enzymes are cooked out.

If your child reacts to this . . .	Try this . . .
Whole milk, cream	Low fat milk, yogurt
Donuts, cake, cookies	Crackers, pretzels bread, pasta, rice, cereal
Fried chicken, hot dogs, sausage, bacon	Breaded chicken, Kosher hot dogs, lean meat rolled up in a bun, sausage crumbles drained on paper towels, Bac-Os.
High fat sandwich meat like bologna, salami	Low fat sandwich meat like oven roasted chicken
Orange juice, citrus juice, soda, coffee, tea	Water, milk, watered down juices such as white grape, apple, pear
Oranges, lemon, pineapples	Pears, apple, banana, papaya
Beans, cabbage, broccoli, onion and foods that cause gas/burping	Potatoes, parsnips, rutabagas, cook beans with epazote or Beano
Green veggies	Yellow and orange veggies
Tomatoes	Try Prelief sprinkles
Spicy food, peppers, garlic, peppermint	Herbs, small amounts of milder spices, flavored salts if your doctor approves
Chocolate	White chocolate MAY be OK

Caffeine is a problem for many people with reflux. Bubbly drinks, too.

Some children find it is better to avoid beverages with meals and only drink liquids between meals. When you put a liquid in the stomach with a solid meal, the liquid tends to bounce around a lot when the stomach churns.

Some parents report that fruit juices are tolerated most of the time but seem to cause tummy aches other times. There was a scientific study that showed the sugar content and type of sugar varies dramatically from brand to brand and month to month as the fruit crop changes. Welch's tries to make their recipes consistent and you may have better luck with their drinks. White grape may be digested better than purple. Sometimes the patterns are very odd and hard to spot.

My in-laws are from another country and have very different ideas about what to feed a baby with a sensitive tummy. I think of avoca-

dos as adult food and they give it to babies. I think of bananas as good for babies and they insist that big, yellow bananas are hard to digest so babies in their country only get the small, red bananas. And I have to admit they were right. Even the yogurt from the Middle Eastern store seems to sit better.

Your older child is bound to push their luck with forbidden foods at friends' houses or at school. It is natural for a child to experiment and try to eat the foods other kids love. She will learn her limits through experience.

Some children with reflux just don't have issues with the foods that bother most gerdlings.

My daughter can just look at a bottle of OJ and start refluxing. On the other hand, she drinks a can of V8 every day- strange behavior in a 2 year old, but that's what her 4-year-old brother drinks. She loves spicy salsa (when she gets tired of dipping the chips, she just lifts up the bowl and drinks it down), and thinks a good snack is 2 or 3 tomatoes. It doesn't aggravate her reflux at all. Caffeine had no apparent impact either.

Nutritional Drinks and Vitamins

Ask the doctor about nutritional supplements such as formula, nutritional drinks, vitamins and minerals. Infants and children who are not eating from all food groups and slow growers may benefit from vitamin and mineral supplements. Keep in mind that vitamins can be harsh on sensitive stomachs. It may take a bit of trial and error to find one that agrees with her sensitive tummy and her sensitive taste buds.

The doctor may keep a toddler on an infant formula beyond age one year and then introduce a nutritional drink for children ages 1-12 years. A vitamin supplement may be used if there are nutritional deficits from a limited diet.

We tried every chewable, gummy, bubble gum vitamin on the shelf and they all caused my daughter to urp and burp. She complained that she could taste the vitamin taste in her mouth and refused to take them. I think she was refluxing the vitamins. We finally stopped trying a chewable vitamin and switched to a pill she could swallow. Now she doesn't complain about taking the vitamins.

Consult a Nutritionist

Many kids who eat a limited variety of foods or have a small appetite still manage to eat a healthy diet and grow well. If you are trying an elimination diet or feeding a picky toddler, you may want to consult with a nutritionist. If your baby or toddler only eats from two food groups, you may want to track her intake over several days and show the list to a nutritionist just to be sure she is getting all the vitamins and nutrients she needs.

A nutritionist with a background in reflux and dealing with picky eaters can offer guidance and strategies. However, many of the standard recommendations for weight gain such as adding calories from butter and half-and-half may backfire with children who have reflux – adding fats often aggravates reflux.

Nutritionists who specialize in working with children who have medical problems often know of formulas that are appropriate for toddlers who are too old for baby formulas but refuse other foods. Your grocery store probably only carries one brand, but there are several more that they can order for you.

Identify Oral Motor and Sensory Issues

If a child receives aggressive medical treatment for reflux but still seems afraid to eat or coughs and chokes when eating, an oral motor or sensory problem may be interfering with eating. A speech or occupational therapist can evaluate your child and identify the cause of the feeding problem. See the section on Feeding Clinics.

Sticking to the Diet Outside the House

While adhering to a special diet may be a vital treatment, it can be frustrating to you and your child. Your child may not appreciate your attempts to monitor the foods he eats at home, school and other situations. It can be embarrassing to be different and this includes eating special food.

Well-meaning adults and young children may not realize how important it is to adhere to a special diet and may try to offer a child "just a bite" of foods that make your child feel bad later. Your job as a parent is to educate all of the people your child interfaces with and provide alternative foods.

Many parents feel a great deal of stress about all of the meal planning, shopping, reading labels and supervision.

> My daughter is on the Everything Free Diet: dairy free, wheat free, eggs free, soy free etc. My doctor taught me to look for kosher pareve labels since anything pareve is dairy free. Also kosher markets, etc will all be able to direct you to dairy free/pareve items.

Celebrate Special Occasions

For most families, food is an important part of holidays and celebrations. It may be disappointing to celebrate a holiday while on a special diet. How do you enjoy a holiday when eating is one of the least pleasurable experiences your child can imagine? But we need to press on and celebrate anyway. It is time to put on your "creativity hat" and develop a new tradition born of necessity.

> Thanksgiving dinner was going just great. My daughter ate all of the white foods - mashed potatoes, roll and a little turkey. She would have blended in with the whole Thanksgiving scene except she couldn't leave the table without letting out one of her world-famous ten second burps!!! Then all of the comments started...

> Halloween, like all holidays can be tough with reflux. My kids stray from the foods and routines that help them manage their reflux and we all have to live with the consequences. In our house, candy can be traded for money or a treat that doesn't aggravate their tummies. We save a bag of Halloween candy to decorate our Christmas gingerbread house - a family tradition.

> We are setting new traditions in our family that are not oriented around food. Instead of candy for the stockings, the children get a few small books. Instead of Easter egg hunting, we have more fun decorating the plastic eggs and hanging them on a tree.

In our house, the kids are allowed to eat as much candy as they want on Halloween night. Then it disappears so we only have one night of bellyaches.

Establish a Routine

Nothing has been the same since the birth of your child. Remember how you used to sit at the table and eat a meal with real dishes and even forks?! While eating a family meal may have gone by the wayside, now is the time to establish a family meal routine.

It is probably not realistic to have every meal together as a family. Try to focus on several meals a week when most family members are together. At your house, this might be breakfast or lunch. Everyone needs to sit at the table together with the TV off.

Adults are watched closely by little eyes whether we like it or not. Our eating habits and attitudes are passed along from adults to children. We set the tone by engaging in pleasant conversation, eating slowly, enjoying ourselves and following a simple routine. Remember to let your child see you trying new foods and eating all of those fruits and vegetables we know they are trying to avoid at all cost.

It is important to limit mealtime to a reasonable amount of time based on your child's age and developmental level. Five or ten minutes for a meal is about as long as a toddler can sit still.

Perhaps it is like a three ring circus in your house at mealtime - someone spills the glass of milk while someone else complains about the menu and the phone rings as you are answering the door. It may take time to establish a routine. Take it slowly. Not every meal will be perfect. Don't make the situation worse by getting upset.

Having dinner together as a family every night was completely impossible – my husband isn't even home until eight many nights. We decided that one evening per week is Family Dinner and Movie Night. We turn off the phones, put on our best PJs, hit three take-out windows in 15 minutes and come back home to have a family date. For us, this is the only way to have a pleasant meal that everybody enjoys.

Check Your Emotions at the Kitchen Door

Feeding your child may have been an unpleasant experience from day one. You may feel tremendous pressure to help your child gain weight, eat nutritious foods and catch up on feeding milestones. It doesn't help that you may get the feeling others blame you for holding your child back and causing the feeding issues. It is easy to put pressure on your child in hopes that she will rise to the occasion. Usually, just the opposite occurs. Just as you put pressure on her, she feels cornered and refuses to eat with even greater will and noisy crying.

Somehow, anger and frustration need to be left at the kitchen door. This can be very difficult if a "meal" consists of five cheerios and a few sips of milk. Or if you just made a meal from scratch and it was soundly rejected by a very harsh food critic, namely your little one sitting in a high chair with a stern look on her face.

> *She is doing well now, but the road has been tough. My daughter went through many stages where she refused to eat. The thing that freaked me out the most was when she would chew her food, then spit it out because she didn't want to swallow it. She figured out that swallowing solids made her hurt, so she would try to avoid it even though she was clearly hungry.*

> *The doctor told me to stop worrying about what and how often she eats. He said kids will eat when they get hungry enough, if we leave them alone about it (Keep in mind my child was in a healthy weight range). Because I was desperate, I tried it. To my amazement, it worked. When it wasn't a battle anymore, she started to eat. It wasn't perfect, but I decided this was going to have to be okay.*

If you find yourself unable to face the mealtime routine, ask someone else to help with mealtime. Perhaps dad can be in charge of a meal and you could go to another room or even leave the house.

Sometimes control over eating is a big issue. A child who is fussy about spoon-feeding may not be complaining about the food, she may want to control the spoon and do the feeding herself. Be sure to give her room for experimenting and independence whenever possible.

It was less messy if I gave my toddler two empty spoons to use as drumsticks and kept one myself for spooning in food. He could play and not get angry that I took his spoon.

Self-feeding can be very messy with 75% of the food ending up worn by the eater and 25% actually getting into the mouth. It may appear that nothing was consumed at all. Cleaning up a terrible, sticky mess can get old rather quickly. Again, it is best to make feeding your gerdling a family affair and let everyone have the pleasure of helping. The good news is all of this messy eating will lead to more independence and more healthy food intake over time.

I have pictures of my son with food in his hair and all over the kitchen. He was a picky eater so I didn't want to stop the fun. He insisted that all finger foods must be dipped in yogurt so it was even messier. We just stripped him to a diaper before putting him in the high chair. When he was done with all the dipping, licking and finger-painting, I hosed him down in the sink with the sprayer and my husband hosed down the high chair out in the back yard. Lots of fun for him and no pressure from us.

Older kids want to assert their independence by making food choices and deciding when and where they will eat. Children who have medical issues often feel that they have no control in their own lives. One of the earliest ways that children learn to assert control is by not eating what their parents want them to eat. Rejecting food might be a way of rejecting all those situations where adults boss them around.

Older children need to learn to select foods that do not cause digestive issues. Just as you help your older child achieve independence in other situations, you want to help her become skilled at listening to her stomach and remembering to use self-control and healthy habits. But she can't learn to make good choices if you don't let her make her own choices – a few mistakes are part of the learning process.

I was surprised when my 11 year old told me she didn't think she should drink soda anymore. I think it was embarrassing to burp really loud and it was making her reflux worse. I asked her what she wanted to drink instead and made a mental note to buy a lot!

Play With Your Food

While you are establishing your mealtime routine, remember to have a little fun. Eating may feel like serious work to both you and your child. Try to keep things light and humorous. Take a look at mealtime from your child's point of view and make sure eating is pleasurable.

Young children love to feed mom or dad. Let your child give you all of the broccoli trees and apple slices she won't touch. Be sure to emphasize how delicious the food is and thank her repeatedly for giving you this delicious food. She will think this is very funny!

> *My daughter loved to share her food more than she liked to eat it. She would put a cracker on my plate, I would pass it to my husband and he would put it back on her plate. Often, she would eat it after it went around the circle a few times. The relatives bought into the game right away and didn't seem to notice that she only ate a little of the holiday dinner. They were focused on the cute sharing, not the lack of eating.*

Some children like having a special plate, cup and utensils featuring their favorite character. Using special plates and cups conveys the message that mealtime is special and yet predictable. Some children feel more secure knowing they can count on the same utensils. Don't worry if you find yourself packing these items for all outings.

Some children thrive on pretend play activities with an eating theme- get out the miniature tea set and feed the teddy bear, doll and all of the neighborhood children. Have a picnic at the park or in your playroom, eat on a rock or on the jungle gym.

> *Our daughter learned about civilized meals by being the hostess, not a guest. Her favorite meal was a tea party so we held semi-formal tea parties where we invited the neighbor girls and dressed up – dolls, too. We used real china plates and wineglasses for our milk. My daughter decided the menu and even took an occasional bite. Sometimes we invited the dog and had him wear a bib.*

Some children respond well to eating with a friend or relative or with other children. A trip out to a restaurant can be very entertaining and distracting during mealtime.

Older children should go food shopping with you and help select a new food now and then. Perhaps they have seen another child eating a food or had a new food while a guest at a friend's house. Hunt for different types of food. Have your child chose one vegetable, one fruit, one meat, etc. You never know what will stimulate a positive association.

> *My extremely picky 4 year old came home from preschool and announced that she tasted 3 kinds of apple during Apple Day and asked me to buy the yellow kind - her new favorite. She also helped make applesauce and announced that it was delicious. I almost passed out from shock. Here was a kid who insisted on the same foods over and over and she ate four new foods at school! It showed me that she was capable of trying new foods despite all of the fussing and complaining she did at home.*

Reading storybooks about eating can be very motivating and instructive. Popular books include: The Very Hungry Caterpillar, Green Eggs and Ham and If you give a Mouse a Cookie. Use the repetitive nature of these books to playfully talk about eating. In Green Eggs and Ham, Sam says, "I do not like green eggs and ham." You can say, "I do not like green eggs and ham, but I do like ham sandwiches. I wonder if Sam would like a ham sandwich just like this one."

Older children may be interested in helping with simple food preparation. It doesn't matter if they eat the food or not, it just gives them an opportunity to touch and smell a food up close.

> *My child became the salad maker of the house. She ripped the lettuce, selected the vegetables and toppings and proudly presented the bowl at the table. Of course, she never did eat any of it!*

> *I went from carrying a diaper bag to a snack bag. My daughter needed to graze all day and sip water in between. I didn't go anywhere without a large tote bag filled with her favorite comfort foods such as dry cereal, crackers, pretzels and a water bottle or juice box. Sometimes we were out longer than we expected or got stuck in traffic. I was so glad that I had my "feed bag" and so was she. Eating frequently really lessened her digestive discomfort and helped her maintain her weight. When it comes to feeding, I have adopted the Boy Scout motto - Be Prepared!!*

◆

Before my daughter was diagnosed with GERD at age 3 years, she showed many unusual eating patterns. She only wanted to nurse in the first year. She wanted to nurse all the time, 24/7. She refused all baby food and eventually just went to table foods that she could pick up and eat herself. We never did the baby food, stages, etc. My daughter was always open to new eating experiences. We did the tea party stage - play with food, eating not mandatory but encouraged. We did the Asian thing - chopsticks and pretty, little bowls and accessories. She found that she loved Chinese take out! We tried every bagel at the neighborhood bagel store (a destination via bike) and she settled on spinach bagels as the hands-down favorite. Yes, we still have stacks of frozen macaroni and cheese in the freezer but we also have some foods that our whole family can live with. It is a continuing journey. We gain some new foods and lose some old ones. Illness or a bad reflux day can be enough to take a food off the "safe" list. It can be very frustrating.

Notes:

17 ADVANCED MEDICAL TOPICS

If your child is not experiencing these types of significant difficulties, there is no need for you to read this chapter. This chapter is for the parents of older children as well as children with very severe reflux or special medical and developmental issues.

You should read this chapter if:

Your child has significant complications from reflux
Your child has multiple health issues
Your child has developmental issues
Your child has unusual symptoms that do not respond to typical treatment

The bottom line is your child is just not getting better despite a medicine cabinet full of medications and endless trips to the doctor and pharmacy.

Medical Complications

Most children grow out of reflux by the time they are two with no damage and no lasting problems. The types of complications in this section are quite rare. We didn't go into as much detail on these concepts in the front of the book because it would have terrified parents of babies who have simple reflux.

Everybody thinks reflux is so simple and easy to treat, but my child had every complication in the book at one time or another. It didn't feel simple to me! If I knew that I was going to have a kid with so many health problems I would have gone to medical school instead of another career!

Esophageal

Children who have acid bouncing up into their esophagus for years may eventually develop ulcers or scaring in the esophagus. This is fairly unusual in children but it does happen occasionally. One concern is that a swollen and raw lower esophageal sphincter may stop contracting properly. This means more acid can leak out and more swelling and rawness can happen. This vicious cycle can be hard to break and often requires aggressive treatment.

Esophageal swelling and ulcers are generally quite painful, but scar tissue is not painful. The most common symptom of scar tissue is that your child chokes when swallowing large bites of food. This is because the scar tissue makes the opening of the esophagus narrow or forms webs across the opening.

If the esophagus is constantly being bathed with acid, the cells may start to change and become more like stomach lining cells, which aren't damaged by acid. The body uses this clever way to make the esophagus lining less delicate, but these hybrid stomach/esophagus cells can sometimes grow out of control after many years of refluxing. The term for the half stomach/half esophageal cells is Barrett's Esophagus or pre-cancer. This is extremely rare in children.

It is extremely rare for a child to develop Barrett's Esophagus, but a few children each year are diagnosed with it. Your doctor may suggest doing an endoscopy every so often to make sure that your child is not one of the unlucky few.

Respiratory

When acid or acid vapors get into the airway, they can damage the protective mucus lining of the airway. When the lining is damaged, bacteria and viruses have an opportunity to get through the protective lining and start an infection. As the body tries to heal the damage from the acid, the tissues can swell. The swelling is part of the healing process, but it can sometimes cause a blockage that keeps bacteria trapped. For instance, when your child gets a bit of acid reflux into her sinuses, the acid damages the mucus lining, the swelling can close off the opening to that sinus and then any bacteria that happens to be in the sinus can start a sinus infection.

When acid and food get refluxed into the lungs, your child can develop pneumonia. Many of us know people who walked around for weeks not knowing they had pneumonia and we have gotten the false impression that it isn't dangerous. Pneumonia is quite serious and can leave scars in the lungs. In most cases, it can be treated quickly and successfully, but children and people with health problems can get in very deep trouble from pneumonia and end up hospitalized for long periods.

The airway and the digestive system communicate with each other. When the esophagus senses that acid is headed toward the airway, it sends out an alarm signal. In some children, the airway goes on red alert and tries to protect itself from the acid. The bronchial tubes in the lungs may narrow in an attempt to prevent acid from reaching the lungs. Narrow bronchial tubes can lead to trouble breathing or an asthma attack.

Another way that the airway tries to protect itself is by closing the epiglottis and the vocal cords. Closing is a good thing and protects the airway from acid during the reflux episode. Unfortunately, sometimes they can lock shut and stay shut after the danger of aspiration has passed. This is called a laryngospasm.

A child who is experiencing a larynospasm usually has a very surprised expression on her face. She won't be able to talk and her lips and chest may move as she tries to gasp for air. She will likely start panicking and so will you. It is best to call 911 even though laryngospasms go away by themselves.

A laryngospasm looks very much like choking and you might be tempted to do the Heimlich Maneuver. A very few children will actually start to turn blue and pass out. A laryngospasm is very scary for the adult and even scarier for the child that it is happening to. The good news is that the epiglottis and vocal cords relax eventually and your child will be able to breathe in a few seconds. Probably the scariest seconds of your life. Call 911 anyhow. You can always call back and tell them not to come when she starts breathing.

Extreme Pain

Most children with reflux function fairly well despite the pain. They go to school, they play and they sleep and eat reasonably well. But some children have extreme pain from their reflux. They can't function well because they are in pain. Some have pain that isn't terribly severe but it never lets up and it wears them down. Other kids experience pain that isn't constant but it is very severe. A few kids have been nearly suicidal because of pain.

Lack of Pain

Some children learn to live with pain so well that they no longer seem to feel pain. Their reflux pain teaches them to ignore pain almost completely. These children can break bones and barely complain. Their high pain tolerance can get them into trouble because they don't let you know when they really need medical attention. They may also stop telling you about their reflux symptoms.

> *Our first baby was a classic refluxer. She was miserable, threw up dozens of times a day and never slept. Our second child was so happy and had such a high pain tolerance that we didn't recognize he had terrible reflux and asthma. He didn't get the treatment he needed because he never complained.*

> *My gerdling taught herself to block pain. She was so good at this that she could have dental work with no Novocaine. We figured out that she refused it because she still had major trust issues.*

Referred Pain

The pain from reflux is usually felt in the esophagus. But pain from digestive organs sometimes feels like it is coming from someplace other than the true source of the pain. When you hurt your leg, you don't feel it in your arm, but pain from that comes from the esophagus can be felt anywhere above the belly button or even in the shoulder joint and shoulder blades. This referred (transferred) pain can cause a lot of confusion.

Nausea

It is uncommon for nausea to be a symptom of reflux but some kids do get nauseated when they have bouts of reflux. Nausea is more likely to be caused by other digestive problem, not reflux. If your child experiences nausea, the doctor will probably check for other digestive problems.

Nauseated or nauseous? Did you know that, "I feel nauseated" is the correct phrase to use? If you say, "I feel nauseous," it means you are making other people around you feel like throwing up. The word nauseous rhymes with obnoxious and has a somewhat similar meaning.

Vomiting Bile

Bile is excreted into the small intestine and helps break down food. If your child is throwing up yellowish mucus, it may be bile and you should tell the doctor. Throwing up bile means that the small intestine is letting food move backwards and up into the stomach.

Bleeding

If the damage to the esophagus is severe, your child could vomit blood. Your doctor needs to know about this right away. Blood in the esophagus can also come out when your child has a bowel movement. If you see stools that look like black coffee grounds or tar, call your doctor. Digested blood in the stool usually smells very foul.

Poor Vitamin Absorption

The medicines used to treat reflux can alter the ability of the body to absorb vitamins properly. Vitamin B12 doesn't absorb as well if there is limited stomach acid. Signs of a B12 deficiency include nausea, diarrhea, poor appetite, tingling or burning sensation in the hands or feet, low energy, depression, memory loss and irritability.

Iron is also more difficult to absorb properly when stomach acid is suppressed. A person who has low iron might feel weak, tired, dizzy, cold and out of breath. The lips and fingernails might look blue and the skin is usually pale.

Dental Damage

Most children with reflux don't have any problems with their teeth. The acid can put holes in the teeth that look different from typical cavities. Acid is more likely to damage the sides of the teeth and the points while typical cavities are worst in the crevasses of the molars. Sealers help, but the acid can sometimes get under the sealers and loosen them. A few children have damage that is so severe it can even look like baby bottle mouth.

Dental work may need to be done in the hospital under anesthesia for children who have a history of choking.

Delayed Milestones

There is a great deal of variability when children learn to use large muscles for sitting, pulling to stand and walking. If your infant has been ill from reflux disease, she might have missed opportunities to learn skills. Your baby may have been held much more than a baby without reflux to reduce crying and allow a favorable position for digestion.

> *My daughter never rolled over as a baby due to the fact that she was always held. But she ended up developing just fine and learned to ride a bike in one day when she was only three!*

Speech and Language Delay

A baby with reflux disease may have a few obstacles in her path to developing speech and language. A baby who is crying in pain 24/7 may miss out on play experiences that help develop language. Some of the muscles used for eating are also used for speech. The lack of practice with eating different foods and textures can slow language development a bit.

Delayed Feeding Skills

Feeding skills may be delayed due to a variety of reason including: inability to eat a variety of foods due to an oral motor issue, lack of readiness or lack of experience. While all of your friends were feeding their babies jar after jar of baby food, you were trying to coax your baby to take just a spoonful.

When to Seek Help

During well baby check ups, your doctor will ask you questions about your baby's skill development. Based on this information, your doctor can determine if skills are developing at the expected pace. Your doctor may determine that further testing is needed.

A Child Find or Early Intervention program is available in most communities and offers free developmental screening and testing for children from birth to age 5 years. Your child will think the testing is just a bunch of fun games, but the examiner is watching her every move closely. You will be given a written report that describes the testing and any recommended treatments.

> *My story: At age two, my gerdling didn't talk much at all. She communicated in gestures and made her wants known very clearly, but not by talking. Child Find did a half-day evaluation and found that she probably just didn't want to talk because it hurt her throat. They told us to stop responding to the gestures for a few days and see how she would react. Not only did she start talking, within a few weeks we were joking that she should have an OFF button.*

Reflux in Special Populations

Reflux disease is extremely common in children with special needs. A child with autism, neurological and muscle tone issues, Down Syndrome or prematurity is more likely to have reflux than typical children. Children with "midline" birth defects of the esophagus, heart, lungs or diaphragm are also highly prone to reflux.

A child with special needs may have a multitude of developmental, behavioral and medical issues so it can be hard to sort out all of the symptoms. Parents report that the reflux is often overlooked and underdiagnosed when there are other issues.

> *My child has multiple medical and development issues and is confined to a wheelchair. He needs help with eating, dressing, bathing and mobility. However, the hardest thing for me is to deal with his reflux. It wakes him and us up at night, it makes him irritable and it makes it hard to feed him.*

Some babies have low muscle tone (hypotonia) or high muscle tone (hypertonia). The muscle tone may affect the digestive system as well as feeding and swallowing. Your child may need more time and patience to progress to textured food and table food. It is important to look for nonverbal cues from your child to determine if she is in pain or having trouble managing the texture or flavor of a new food. It can be scary to choke, so it is important to go slowly when starting a new food.

Reflux is extremely common in babies born early. A baby born prematurely may also have feeding and digestive issues due to an immature neurological system, medications, breathing issues and an immature digestive system. A premature baby may need special feeding assistance from an occupational therapist, speech therapist and nutritionist. Reflux is so common in preemies that doctors often just assume they have it. It used to be common to give all preemies medication for reflux. Now we know better – preemies can have more side effects and problems with medications.

About 50-70% of children with Down Syndrome have reflux symptoms. Children with Down Syndrome have low muscle tone, which can cause the lower esophageal sphincter to open more easily, allowing acid to reflux upward into the esophagus. Many children with Down Syndrome have difficulty with feeding since the low muscle tone also affects sucking and swallowing.

Reflux disease is extremely common in children with autism. However, it may be difficult to sort out the symptoms since many children with autism also have extreme food preferences (only eat green food, only eat crunchy food), as well as sensory processing issues. In addition, communication may be significantly affected, leading to poor communication of wants and needs (hunger, pain, request food, end a meal). You may find that it takes a great deal of trial and error to find some "safe" foods as well as to find a dose of medication that controls pain.

> *My son with autism developed intense, frequent temper tantrums at age 3. His doctor prescribed an antidepressant to control his outbursts. I felt really uncomfortable about this and called his Pediatric Gastroenterologist because he still had mild reflux symptoms after stopping his reflux meds a few months ago. We decided to try a dose of reflux medication for two weeks to see if this would help the reflux and the behavior. I was amazed to see him transform almost immediately. He still had occasional tantrums, but he slept and ate better and best of all, he said three new words.*

Looks Like Reflux But It's Not

There are many reasons for vomiting. If your child does not respond to typical treatments, has multiple symptoms or has odd symptoms, you and your doctor may consider whether you child could have another disease with symptoms that look like reflux.

In medical school, the saying goes, "If you hear hoof beats, think horses. There are many horses but few zebras." It means, before considering an exotic or rare illness, don't overlook a common diagnosis. So a "zebra" in medical slang is a rare or unusual medical problem. Doctors are cautioned not to immediately consider a rare condition before looking at the possibility of common medical problem. But after considering the common explanations, it may be time to look at the rare possibilities.

Some conditions to look at if you are zebra hunting:

Lactose Intolerance
Fructose Intolerance
Milk / Soy Protein Intolerance
Gastroparesis (delayed gastric emptying)
Helicobactor Pylori
Gall bladder, liver or pancreatic dysfunction
Eosinophilic Diseases
Autonomic Dysfunction, (Dysautonomia, Postural Orthostatic Tachycardia, Neurally Mediated Hypotension, Orthostatic Intolerance, Neutrally Mediated Syncope, vagus nerve dysfunction)
Pyloric Stenosis / Pyloric Spasms
Achalasia / Dysphagia
Tracheomalacia or Laryngomalacia
Celiac Disease (Gluten Intolerance)
Cyclic Vomiting Syndrome
Immune Deficiency diseases
Mitochondrial Disorders
Metabolic Diseases
Vocal Cord Dysfunction
Chronic Intestinal Pseudo Obstruction
Prader Willi Syndrome
Alkaline Reflux / Bile Reflux
Irritable Bowel Syndrome (IBS)
Reactions to medications
Mastocytosis
Abdominal angioedema
Hypochlorhydria
Tyrosinemia

Doing your own research

If you are searching for advanced medical information, you might want to ask a librarian for help. Most librarians are very good at finding information for people who need to learn about medical problems. Start with a community librarian and ask for a referral to a medical librarian if you have trouble finding what you need. Many county library systems have at least one medical librarian. Libraries may also subscribe to medical web sites that are expensive.

Some medical libraries let the public use their resources. Try the one at your local hospital or a medical school. These libraries also have text books which can provide overviews of the diseases you are researching. Textbooks are often the best source of "differential diagnosis" lists.

When you doing your own searches on the internet, try using several different search engines. What you get from Yahoo is very different from what you get with Google. And there are search engines like Dog-Pile that pull up results from Yahoo, Google and many others all at the same time.

When you find something interesting on the internet, save it! You may never find it again.

> *My story: When Katie was little, I did some research on autonomic instability. She had a few symptoms and so did a friend's child, but it didn't seem like a perfect match. It wasn't until years later that the information proved more useful. It turns out that autonomic symptoms often get worse as kids start to hit puberty and get taller. Both of the girls were diagnosed in their teens when their symptoms got worse. Autonomic instability is probably the real reason that both girls had terrible GERD.*

Internet searches are based on key words and combinations. Make a list of your child's symptoms and try using several in combination. You may have the best luck by focusing on the symptoms that don't really fit for reflux such as nausea. Have other people review the list of symptoms and do searches for you – they are likely to use different search criteria and find completely different information. If you aren't getting anywhere with looking up your child's symptoms, look up the symptoms of the diseases listed above and do your search backwards.

My son was being treated for reflux and he kept getting worse and worse. He was finally admitted to the hospital and seen by every specialist there. Nobody could figure out what was wrong. I wrote a summary of his medical issues and sent copies to everybody I could think of. Finally, somebody came up with the answer – he was having a serious reaction to the Reglan.

Many web sites and books can help you with your search for a mystery diagnosis. "Symptom checker" sites and sites dedicated to helping find a "missed diagnosis" can be very helpful.

On great thing to look for online is lessons on how to find reputable medical information online. A search with these key words will give you the scoop on avoiding bad information and sites that want to sell you a miracle cure.

Doctors sometimes feel that parents who do a lot of medical research are just overreacting. But sometimes Dr. Mom is correct. Remember to frame your conversation with the doctor so you don't come across as overbearing or bossy. Listen to your doctor's point of view and assessment of the symptoms you are worried about. YOU: The Smart Patient: An Insider's Handbook for Getting the Best Treatment, by Michael F. Roizen and Mehmet C. Oz has lots of good information about working with your doctor to solve a medical mystery.

Advanced Treatment: Feeding Programs

A feeding clinic runs intensive programs for children who won't or can't eat. These clinics are often run by the gastroenterology or developmental departments of a local hospital. Some happen to be located in hospitals that work only with children who have serious developmental delays but their feeding teams also work with children who are neurologically normal. There are a few freestanding clinics, often run by speech therapists. Some programs are so intense that the children and parents stay overnight.

When you look at feeding programs, pay particular attention to the philosophy and methods they use. There are drastic differences from one program to another. Some programs work with children who are still in pain and other clinics want to be assured the pain is gone before they start their work.

251

Feeding therapy can be very intense but very helpful. You may be asked to practice exercises and activities at home and come to a clinic weekly or monthly. Since mothers are often the ones bringing the children to feeding therapy and implementing the plan at home, it is easy to burn out. Involve other family members and friends in the process as much as possible.

If you are considering a feeding program, you might want to check programs all over the country. If you are staying overnight for a whole week, you might as well travel to find the program that is the best fit for your child's particular feeding issues.

Advance Treatment: Tube Feeding

You may have heard about tube feeding as a possible feeding method for an infant who is isn't able to eat enough by mouth. Tube feeding may be a last resort method of providing nourishment. While tube feeding increases intake, it can also overfill the stomach and increase reflux and vomiting.

A nasogastric (NG) tube is a thin flexible tube that is inserted into the nose and down into the stomach. A syringe may be attached to the tube and liquid nutrition such as breast milk or formula is poured into the tube and directly into the stomach, bypassing the mouth.

Because the tube can be irritating to your baby, it is generally used as a short-term feeding intervention during an acute illness or feeding problem. If it is determined that a tube feeding is needed for a longer period, a gastrostomy tube (G-tube) may be recommended.

A G-tube is installed surgically. It is a short tube that runs from the outside of the belly, through the abdominal wall and straight into the stomach. It is securely attached on the inside and the outside. A small incision is made into the wall of the stomach and a thin, flexible gastrostomy tube is inserted. The incision heals quickly. When the tube is no longer needed for venting or nutrition, it can be taken out and the small hole will usually close on it's own in a few weeks.

Liquid nutrition and medications can be poured down a large syringe (called a bolus feeding) or a feeding pump can be attached to the tubing so that formula can be dripped into the stomach at a predetermined rate and speed.

The outside of the tube may have a clamp or it may have a closure (called a button) that looks a bit like the cover on the nozzle of an inflatable pool toy. A button is very small and not as bulky as having a tube hanging under the clothing at all times.

> I had done everything I could to feed my daughter and I was exhausted from the effort. Although, it was a hard decision, I finally agreed to tube feeding. The tube helped her grow and have the strength to start feeding therapy.

Check with the doctor before putting any medicine in a feeding tube (gastrostomy or nasogastric tube) and follow instructions carefully. Sometimes the tubing becomes clogged or thick medication sticks to the walls of the tubing. The doctor may have to speak to the manufacturer of the tube of the mediations to get directions.

Advanced Treatment: Surgery

The surgery is called a fundoplication. It involves wrapping the upper part of the stomach around the base of the esophagus to make a one-way valve, which prevents reflux. It is a major surgery and often has a significant recovery period.

The Nissan Fundoplication is the most common type of reflux surgery for children in the United States. Some surgeons prefer to use the Thal or Toupet techniques when they do fundoplications. Your surgeon will choose the technique that works best for them.

Many surgeons have been trained to perform the surgery laparoscopically. A laparoscope is a camera that allows the surgeon to see inside the abdomen without making a large opening. The surgeon makes several tiny cuts and inserts the camera and instruments through these holes. This is often called "band aid surgery" because the patient has such small incisions that a band-aid can cover the stitches. One of the big advantages is that recover time is usually shorter than traditional surgery. A traditional "open" surgery may be necessary for a very small infant or for other reasons.

There are several other procedures in use for adults, which can stop reflux. They are not true "surgical" procedures because the surgeon makes the esophagus into a one-way valve without cutting. They are done using an endoscope in the esophagus. The Stretta, EndoCinch, Bard, Plicator and Gatekeeper are not currently available for children. Many insurance companies will not cover these procedures. Some surgeons are experimenting with a true fundoplication that is done though the esophagus rather than through the abdominal wall.

Considering Surgery

It is important to remember that surgery is an uncommon treatment for reflux disease and is used only for a small number of cases. Many parents worry needlessly about the surgery when it is not even indicated.

Doctors and surgeons have different reasons for recommending a surgical procedure to treat GERD. Reasons for surgery may include one or more of the following:

Esophagitis
Apnea
Failure to thrive
Pneumonia
Asthma
Airway damage
Strictures
Barrett's Esophagus
Apparent Life Threatening Events - ATLE's
Medicines don't provide relief
Significant pain
Significant oral motor disorders
The reflux isn't going away after several years of adequate medication

Surgery may not be beneficial if there is:

Significant delayed gastric emptying
A significant motility issue in the esophagus or intestines
A significant allergic basis to the reflux

The medical team and the family will usually exhaust every treatment option before considering a surgical procedure for gastroesophageal reflux. The doctor and surgeon will want to rule out other conditions that may impact the success of the surgery such as delayed gastric emptying, food allergies and diseases that look like reflux.

Your family may decide that you can handle all the extra work of special meals, night waking, medications, etc to avoid surgery. Other families find that chronic pain coupled with extra caretaking makes surgery look like an option worth considering. Some families are nervous about the long-term use of powerful medications.

As parents, we are programmed to help our children avoid anything unpleasant and the thought of surgery is very scary. On the other hand, a few parents may feel a sense of relief that a surgical procedure may be able to "fix" the problem and decrease their child's pain and the extra work related to reflux.

Books, the web and other information sources can provide everything from a tutorial on how to do the procedure to medical journal articles and more. It is important to ask questions and receive a full explanation of the surgery. A few children have a very rocky recovery, and their parents often feel terrible. It is emotionally helpful to know that you made the decision very carefully.

Parents who want to research the medical literature for information about the surgery and the success rate are faced with hundreds of studies and many, many different criteria for "success." One study may look at quality of life as criteria for success while others will look at need for medication, return of symptoms, decrease in cough and asthma, pH levels before and after surgery or endoscopy results. Be sure to ask the surgeon for information on outcomes and risks.

This surgery requires a great deal of skill and practice. For the best results, try to find a surgeon who has done this exact procedure many times.

Questions to Ask the Doctor

Parents will have many questions about the indications for surgery as well as about the procedure.

Is the reflux causing damage that is not reversible?

Is the reflux causing life-threatening symptoms?

Is there an immediate need for surgery or is there time to explore options?

Have all medications and combinations been thoroughly explored?

What is known now about the long-term affects of the medications?

Is my child young enough that the reflux can still be expected to resolve?

Are we 100% sure this is reflux?

Have there been contradictory test results?

Have other conditions that cause reflux symptoms been fully ruled out?

What do you think will happen without the surgery?

Have you done this exact surgery before? On a child like mine? How many? What was the outcome? How do you rate success?

If your child has had multiple surgeries, ask about the new techniques for preventing adhesions.

Scary Surgery Stories on the Internet

Reflux surgery is fairly common and has a good track record for success. However, there are many scary stories floating around the web about fundoplication surgery to treat reflux. It may even seem that it is hard to find a story with a happy ending.

It is important to consider that all surgical procedures carry some risk ranging from mild, temporary symptoms to a worsening of the medical condition. For some children, it can be a life saving procedure. For others, it can be a cure, allowing a child to grow and develop without long term consequences.

The reality is, most children benefit from the surgery and have a good outcome. The parents of the kids who had successful surgery are not staying up late to post their story on an internet discussion board. These parents are sleeping all night and enjoying the web to register their now healthy kids for the soccer team and recovering from a difficult season of parenthood. Occasionally, they will admire the surgical scars as a distant reminder of their former lives, now faded and faint. We seldom hear their stories.

After the Surgery

In the hospital, your child will be given strong pain relief and an IV for nourishment. As she feels better, pain medication will be decreased and food intake will begin. First, clear liquids and soft food are introduced since the esophagus will be swollen and choking may occur.

Be sure to stay in the hospital until you and your child feel ready to come home and eat and drink enough to stay hydrated. Most children need to restrict their activities for a few weeks and slowly increase their diet to more solid foods. Most children are back to a normal diet in a few days, but it is not uncommon for this to take a few months.

Your child may have a gastrostomy tube placed during the surgery for releasing (called venting) air from the stomach or if there is a history of feeding aversion or nutrition issues.

In the days and week following surgery, your child might experience gas bloat, which is a build up of air in the stomach. This will feel very uncomfortable to your child because she will probably not be able to burp. Decrease gas bloat by avoiding fizzy drinks, eating slowly and chewing thoroughly. If your child has a tube, it can be opened briefly during and after meals to release the air.

A few children develop dumping syndrome. The food dumps rapidly into the intestines instead of going in at a slow pace. The rapid release of stomach contents into the intestines produces strong nausea often accompanied by sweating, weakness and diarrhea. It can be treated.

Adhesions are bands of scar tissue that cause the walls of the stomach to stick to other nearby organs. This is a rare complication of any abdominal surgery that becomes more likely when a child has multiple abdominal surgeries. Symptoms include not passing stool, extreme cramping pain, bloating and dehydration.

Because your child won't be able to vomit, it is important to avoid food poisoning and to keep all poisons locked up. If your child eats something poisonous, you will need to go to the emergency room right away.

If Your Child is Hospitalized

Most children with reflux never end up in the hospital. Even most of the testing can be done on an outpatient basis. But some of our little gerdlings end up needing surgery and some seem to catch every bug that comes within miles.

There are plenty of wonderful books on how to handle hospitalizations. This info is just a sampling but you may not have enough advanced warning to do any other reading,

Ask the doctors how long they think you will be in the hospital. Make a contingency plan for twice as long as they are guessing.

The day you are admitted, get on the phone and ask for these things:
Child life visit
Chaplain visit
Social worker to help make connections to services outside the hospital
A laptop, a cordless phone, books, movies and a DVD player – often Child Life has them to loan to families.
The introduction book that every hospital has for parents – it has the cafeteria hours, location of the family library and lots of other important info.

Arrange for two visitors every day. They should call the room or the nurses desk right before leaving home to be sure you are not about to go to another part of the hospital for a test.

Start a notebook. By the third day, you will have way too many details running around in your head to keep them straight. If mom and dad are taking turns staying at the hospital, this notebook can help you make sure you both have every detail you might need when your spouse is home asleep or in the shower.

You have the right to be as involved as you want in your child's care. When the doctors do "rounds" every morning, you are allowed to be present and participate in the discussion.

> *I was always afraid I would miss talking to the doctors if I slipped out to the parent lounge to get a shower. I put a big note on my daughter's door that said, "Don't do rounds without mom!"*

Write the name of each doctor, nurse, technician, etc. Write the name of each test and the results. Who called or visited each day and what they brought – especially if it was something like a movie that you need to give back to them later. List the medicines, dosages and when they are given. List who you called – did you call the primary care doctor and the insurance company? Even list the name of the pet sitter.

Be very nice to the staff. You can even bring a basket of candy and put it at the nurses' station. Do you want more people to visit the room and keep you company? Keep a candy dish in the room and let the staff know you want more visitors.

Hospitals are not the cleanest places in the world. You won't find any dirt in them, but the battle to keep down the germs is constant. There is a reason that each patient has their own stethoscope, blood pressure cuff and tourniquet. Be extra careful of hygiene to be sure you don't catch anything in the hospital. If your child drops a pillow on the floor, ask for a new case. Watch closely to be sure that nobody puts a piece of medical tape on the bed rail and then puts it on your child's IV. Keep your toothbrush in a case.

Deciding to Have Another Child

After having one baby with reflux, many weary parents are sure they would never have the stamina to risk bringing another baby with reflux into their family. There is no firm data on how likely your chances are. Researchers who are studying families that have a strong history of reflux say that it appears your chances of having a second child with reflux are strongest if your child is much sicker than the typical child with reflux.

> *It is such a tough decision. A good friend of mine decided not to have another one. I decided to take the chance and now I have a 6 week old with bad reflux. Honestly sometimes I regret my decision. Even if you have been through this before and know what to do, it is still hard at night when you get no sleep, hard to watch your baby suffer and think it your fault.*

◆

Make your GI appointments when you are 8 months pregnant!

259

◆

It is really hard the second time around, I will be honest. But there is a difference in that you do know it will end someday and that kind of gets you through the day.

◆

I knew what was happening and marched right in to the doctor to begin treatment.

◆

We were told that reflux was not genetic but at five days of age, I knew that our new baby was just like our first. I looked at my husband and said, "It's Back!"

◆

I personally think in many ways it is easier the next time around because you are more knowledgeable and know how to help your hurting baby. It's the parents who have a perfect baby first who are in for rough a ride when their second is a refluxer.

Munchausen Syndrome by Proxy

Munchausen Syndrome by Proxy (MSBP) is a rare type of child abuse in which caregivers, usually mothers, fabricate illnesses or make their children sick in an attempt to draw attention to themselves and seek sympathy from the medical community.

There is a lot of confusion about whether Munchausen Syndrome by Proxy is a psychiatric diagnosis or just a type of child abuse. The American Psychiatric Association does not recognize the diagnosis, yet there are frequent reports in the media. Many states refuse to use this diagnosis because it is too poorly defined and controversial.

It is known that some parents will harm their children and this child abuse needs to be identified and stopped to protect the children. However, there is a climate of suspicion in the medical community leading some doctors to believe that any child who does not respond to treatment or presents with unusual symptoms may be the victim of Munchausen Syndrome by Proxy. This climate of suspicion is unusually strong in the field of pediatric gastroenterology.

Unfortunately, reflux has many typical and not so typical symptoms as well as symptoms that change over time. Seldom does a doctor see what you experience at home. Doesn't it seem that the baby always sleeps during the entire doctor's visit while you are describing in vivid detail hours of crying and vomiting from midnight until 6am?

My heart sinks when I get the occasional call from a mother telling me the baby was taken away by protective services and the mother is under investigation because the doctor thinks she was lying. When I talk to these mothers, they usually tell me about symptoms that are unusual but fully within the spectrum of reflux. I believe most of these cases stem from poor communication and a lack of understanding of the enormous burden of care required by a baby with severe reflux.

I can understand how a doctor might be concerned about the unusual symptoms, but I wish there was a better understanding of how complex some of these kids can be. Perhaps there is a better way of addressing odd symptoms without blaming the mother. A mother who is frantic and asking the doctor to do tests or "fix" the reflux is just trying to advocate for her baby who is suffering. Interpreting this as a desire for unnecessary medical treatment is not helpful.

I am particularly concerned about social workers who are being asked to make medical judgments without medical or psychiatric training. In some cases, judgments have been made without fully examining both the mother and the child and without considering all possible causes for the symptoms. Any child with mystery symptoms or symptoms that don't respond to treatment, needs to be seen by another doctor until a workable treatment or a new diagnosis is found.

This type of allegation rips apart families, causes deep psychological wounds to all family members and extreme financial hardship. Often, the mother is found not guilty, but there are huge long-term consequences to the child and the family.

When you have a suspicious doctor is there truly ANYTHING you can do or evidence that you can provide to them that would look like anything other than Munchausen's Syndrome by Proxy? The quote "thou doest protest too much" comes to mind. The more you try to prove you are right the more red flags go up to an already suspicious doctor. In fact, all of the things you do to advocate for your child-getting copies of tests, writing a history, learning the lingo and getting all kinds of specialists could simply serve to reinforce doctor's suspicions. It is tough to know where to draw the line.

Notes:

18 INTEGRATIVE, ALTERNATIVE AND COMPLEMENTARY MEDICINE

Alternative and complementary techniques are becoming more and more common in the treatment of a variety of problems including reflux disease. This chapter provides just a brief overview. As with any medical treatment, please be an educated medical consumer. Do your research, use common sense and work with an experienced practitioner.

There has been limited research regarding the safety and effectiveness of alternative and complementary treatments. Practitioners and patients have many of individual success stories regarding specific treatments, but the techniques are often very difficult to study.

What are Complementary and Alternative Treatments?

Complementary and alternative treatment encompasses a variety of treatments and remedies. Many are very old and traditional, often practiced and studied extensively in other countries.

> *"Complementary" tends to refer to treatments that are used along with standard medical care while "alternative" treatments replace standard medical treatment. Integrative medicine is a term used by practitioners who believe that different therapies can be used at the same time and do not in any way compete. Integrative pain management practitioners may use many forms of pain control including pain medicines if needed.*

One of the best sources of information is the National Center for Complementary and Alternative Medicine (NCCAM), part of the National Institutes of Health (NIH). The mission of NCCAM is to: explore complementary and alternative healing practices in the context of rigorous science; train complementary and alternative medicine researchers; and disseminate authoritative information to the public and professionals.

Finding a Practitioner

With any treatment, traditional and non-traditional, it is important to find a practitioner with training and experience with young children. A referral from a friend or other medical professional can be very helpful.

Many practicing MDs and nurses are receiving training in treatments that are not covered in US medical schools. So, it may be possible to find an acupuncturist or hypnotist who has a medical degree too.

Keep your Doctor in the Loop

Be sure to tell your doctor about all other treatments, remedies and even vitamins you are giving your baby or child. Chances are that your pediatrician is used to having patients use complementary medicine. Use this opportunity to educate each other and build trust.

> *Our pediatrician was not very excited when we took our daughter to a hypnotist. But there was no arguing with the success and the doctor called me a few months later to get the name of the hypnotist for another patient.*

Doing Your Homework

Before starting any treatment, weigh the risks and benefits. There are questions to ask yourself and your practitioner:

What are the risks of the treatment?
What are the benefits of the treatment?
Is there research to support the effectiveness of this method with this disease or similar diseases?
Is it possible to blend this treatment with traditional and standard medical care?
What is the recommended length of treatment?
What is the cost?
Is the cost covered by insurance?

When you investigate alternative and complementary treatments, you are unlikely to find a study using the exact technique for children with reflux. But you might be able to find a study of that technique in adults with a similar digestive problem like Irritable Bowel Syndrome. There are few studies so you may have to use common sense and look at studies of diseases that have some overlap with reflux.

Manipulative Techniques

Massage therapy, chiropractic, cranio sacral therapy and physical therapy are called bodywork or manipulative therapies. They involve the practitioner moving the patient's body in specific ways. Acupuncture and acupressure are somewhat different but also involve the practitioner treating the patient's body.

A chiropractor uses manipulation to align the spine and restore health. Practitioners of chiropractic medicine often cite spinal misalignment during birth as a common cause of reflux in newborns. There have been a few reports of serious injury with chiropractic and cranio sacral therapy. Please be very cautious.

I've used a chiropractor through my pregnancy and since my son was 2 weeks old. He was diagnosed with reflux at 5weeks. Chiropractic care did not "cure" him, but I would notice that he was calmer and spit up less after adjustments.

◆

Our son used to scream and vomit 12+ hours a day. No meds seemed to help him and I had several people suggest a chiropractor as they all "knew" someone that it had helped. After 8 months of this, I decided to give it a try. I knew a chiropractor personally who specialized in children so I went to her fully prepared to walk out if she did anything that I didn't approve of with an infant. She used a little pogo stick gadget and worked mainly on his spine between his ribs and his neck. It felt very gentle like a finger tapping. She also cupped her hand and placed it on his stomach to gently manipulate the diaphragm supporting the stomach and lungs. After the first visit, he slept for about 3 hours during the day with no vomiting or tears for 4 hours. We kept going and went 3 times a week for the first 2 months, then 2 times a week for a month, weekly for a month and then had a couple of monthly visits. It wasn't cheap but the first couple of months there was a marked improvement after every visit, then the improvement seemed to slow but he ended up that the only time he vomited was with asthma, tonsillitis, ear infections etc which we were more than happy with. A good chiropractor that specializes in children should be more than happy to listen to your concerns and should explain every step that he/she is taking and why. It was so strange to hear this child laugh through every gentle manipulation instead of the usual uncontrollable tears. It may not work for everyone but we had very good results, we were at the stage that surgery was a very real option.

Cranial Sacral Therapy

Cranial Sacral Therapy is related to chiropractic care. It has been used to treat babies and adults with digestive problems. The theory is that misalignment of the skull bones can pinch the nerves and the spinal cord as they exit the base of the skull. It is believed that gently manipulating the skull bones can relieve pressure on the nerves.

Massage

Infant massage may be used to calm a fussy, irritable baby and reduce digestive discomfort. A certified infant massage therapist may work with an individual baby or provide classes to train parents. There is a specific technique for improving intestinal motility and another for lifting the diaphragm gently to relieve a hiatal hernia.

He seems much more relaxed after the massage and even took a two-hour nap rather than his usual short, fitful catnap.

Acupuncture

Acupuncture is an ancient treatment from China. Small, thin needles are placed on key points on the body to treat a variety of ailments including nausea. Even mainstream medical societies like the American Academy of Pediatrics are hosting lectures on this technique. Acupuncture has proven effective for treating nausea in medical studies.

A few years ago, I was at a medical conference where they gave a demonstration of acupuncture. We were each given a needle that was thinner than a human hair. The lecturer told showed us a specific spot on the shin and told us to use the needle if we wanted. A very light tap on the end of the needle was all it took. Many people in the audience felt immediate nausea. He had deliberately told us a spot that he would never use on a patient because he wanted us to understand the power of this treatment. Then he told us how to cure the nausea using another spot.

Acupressure

Acupressure is similar to acupressure. The points on the body are pressed with the finders or blunt objects instead of using needles. Reflexology is the use of pressure points in the hands or the feet to stimulate other parts of the body. This technique also has a good reputation for nausea.

Alternative Medications

Practitioners of Homeopathic Medicine, Herbal Medicine, Traditional Chinese Medicine, Ayurvedic medicine and Naturopaths and Nutritionists give medications that are not on the FDA drug list.

There is a great deal of concern about contaminated medications and herbs, especially those imported from other countries. Be very careful to work with a practitioner who is concerned about safety.

Homeopathic Medicine

Homeopathy is a system for treating illnesses by giving diluted substances that stimulate the body to recover. For example, nux vomica taken in full strength will induce vomiting, but when diluted to one part per million using a special technique, it can teach the body to reduce vomiting. Remedies are selected based on specific symptoms and patterns, not based on the "cause" of the illness. Side effects are rare but can occur, particularly when overusing the most dilute (strongest) formulations. Homeopathy is very popular in England and Sweden. It is also used in veterinary medicine, so the placebo effect can't fully explain how it works.

Naturopathic Medicine

A Naturopath provides a variety of treatment including diet, vitamins, chiropractic treatments, acupuncture, massage, lifestyle counseling and traditional Chinese medication. The focus is on teaching the body to heal itself.

> *My 15-month-old son had severe croup and painful reflux. I tried everything the doctors told me to do and he just wasn't getting better. One doctor even suggested surgery. At that point, I started seeing a naturopath. Through testing and treatment, my son showed remarkable improvement.*

Herbal Medicine

There are several categories of herbals that may be useful for the treatment of reflux: carminatives soothe the stomach and decrease gas and demulcents offer a protective barrier for irritated tissue. Herbs with antispasmodic properties are often used for digestion.

According to an article in Contemporary Pediatrics (August 2005), many of the common herbal remedies for digestive complaints are classified by the FDA as "Generally Regarded as Safe," or GRAS. Gripe water (made from dill, fennel, or ginger) for colic is the most commonly used herbal remedy for babies. This article also describes a randomized, double bind, placebo controlled study demonstrating that a specific herbal tea eliminated colic in 57% of babies.

It is extremely important to work with an herbal medicine specialist with experience helping infants and young children. Always inform your pharmacist and doctor about any remedies you are using to avoid harmful side effects from other treatments. Herbal medicines may be dangerous, even in small quantities, and may interact with each other or with medications.

Every year there are reports in the news about contaminated herbs. Be sure to ask an experienced practitioner how to choose trustworthy brands or learn how to make your own remedies from high quality ingredients.

Probiotics

Probiotics are beneficial bacteria found in the stomach. Some types of probiotics such as acidophilus, lactobacillus and bifid bacterium may reduce digestive issues such as colic and diarrhea. Some brands of yogurt contain live bacteria. Some baby food manufacturers are starting to add probiotics and "pre-biotics" which are like vitamins for the good bacteria and encourage them to thrive.

Supplements are available as a powder, liquid or pill supplements. There is a trend toward adding bifid bacteria to commercially made baby formula since there is some evidence that this bacteria has beneficial properties for babies with digestive problems.

Digestive Enzymes

Digestive enzymes break down food for absorption and digestion. The body naturally produces digestive enzymes and some are found in the foods we eat. If the digestive system isn't producing enzymes in the correct quantities, symptoms similar to reflux can arise. Fresh papaya and papaya supplements are thought to aid digestion.

> *While we were visiting my mom, she insisted we take my baby to her doctor. Mom's doctor suggested digestive enzymes and they worked like a charm. We tried to take her off them but her reflux would come right back. As long as we keep giving them, she is symptom free.*

Mind-Body Techniques

Biofeedback, Progressive Muscle Relaxation, meditation, yoga, guided imagery, Tai chi, Qui gong, Autogenic Training, Lamaze breathing and hypnosis are all mind-body techniques that can be used to increase relaxation and reduce discomfort/pain.

Children often learn relaxation techniques very quickly. Some pain doctors are using fun video games to teach kids how to do things like relax their neck muscles to reduce headaches. One integrative medicine doctor calls them "video games for your body." Kids learn skills like lowering the temperature of their hand quicker than adults.

Medicine meets Spirituality

Religion and spiritual beliefs can contribute to healing and maintaining a positive outlook on life so that the disease doesn't overwhelm your whole life. Some people find comfort in organized religion and rituals, while others simply seek unstructured ways to feel connected with the universe. Many in the medical profession have stories about patients whose beliefs had a huge impact on their illness.

In the face of adversity, some people turn to their faith as a way of coping while others turn away because disease and illness feel too much like punishment. There are many good books and pastoral counselors who can help if illness is affecting your beliefs.

Notes

RESOURCES

Books and Booklets

Allergy Cooking with Ease
Nicolette Dumke
Starburst Publishing, 2001

The Attachment Parenting Book
Bill and Martha Sears
Little Brown and Company, 2001

The Baby Book
Bill and Martha Sears
Little Brown & Company, 1993

The Breastfeeding Book
Martha Sears, RN
Little Brown & Company, 2000

Breastfeeding Your Baby with Reflux
Laura Barmby
La Leche League International Publications

Colic Solved
Bryan Vartabedian
Ballantine, 2007

Coping with Chronic Heartburn
Elaine Fantle Shimberg
St. Martin's Griffin, 2001

Digestive Wellness
Elizabeth Lipski, MS, CCN.
Keats Publishing, 1999

The Family Nutrition Book
Bill and Martha Sears
Little Brown and Company, 2005

The Fussy Baby Book
Bill and Martha Sears
Little Brown and Company, 1996

Going to School with Acid Reflux
PAGER Association, 2004
From www.reflux.org

Gut Reactions
Raphael Kellman and Carol Colman
Broadway Books, 2002

The Happiest Baby on the Block
Harvey Karp, MD
Bantam Books, 2002

How to Get Your Baby to Sleep
Bill and Martha Sears
Little Brown and Company, 2002

Is This Your Child?
Doris Rapp, MD
Harper Paperbacks, 1992

Infant Massage
Mary Ady, CIMI
www.littlelocalcelebrity.com

Just Take a Bite
Lori Ernsperger and Tania Stegen-Hanson
Future Horizons, 2005.

Life on the Reflux Rollercoaster
Roni MacLean and Jean McNeil
www.infant-reflux.com

Making Life Better for a Child with Acid Reflux
Mike and Tracy Davenport
Sportwork, Inc. 2006

Milk Soy Protein Intolerance Guidebook/Cookbook
Tamara Field, 2001

Nighttime Parenting: How to get Your Baby and Child to Sleep
Bill and Martha Sears
Le Leche League International Book, 1999.

Poor Eaters - Helping Children who Refuse to Eat.
Joel Macht, PhD
Perseus Publishing, 1990.

Secrets of the Baby Whisperer: How to calm, connect, and communicate
with your baby
Tracy Hoggs
Atria Books, 2005.

Tummy Trouble, Funny Tummy, My Endoscopy Story by Jack and
Korky the Kanagroo has a pH Probe
Available from TAP Pharmaceutical Products Inc.
www.prevakids.com

Products - Feeding

Dr. Brown's Natural Flow Bottle
800-778-9001
info@handi-craft.com

Controlled Flow ™ Baby Feeder
800-551-7096
www.bionix.com

Haberman Feeder
Available from many sources: See www.mandyhaberman.com

Mealtimes Catalog - New Visions Feeding Program
800-606-7112
www.new-vis.com

MediBottle and PaciFeeder
888-373-BABY
714-357-6777
www.savi.com

Products - Positioning

Amby Baby Motion Bed
952-974-5100
866-516-baby
www.ambybaby.com
info@ambybaby.com

AR Pillow, Inc
917-699-0608
www.arpillow.com
info@arpillow.com

Comfort Lift Bed
361-767-1888
refluxpillow@yahoo.com

Guardian Sleeper
800-577-5675
www.guardiansleeper.com

Pollywog Nursing Positioner
866-332-0958
www.pollywogbaby.com

Tucker Sling
888-236-9275
info@tuckerdesigns.com
www.tuckerdesigns.com

Patient Support and Information

The Sibling Support Project
A Kindering Center program
206-297-6368
www.siblingsupport.org

Allergy and Asthma Network/Mothers of Asthmatics
800-878-4403
www.aanma.org

American Partnership for Eosinophilic Disorders
713-498-8216
www.apfed.org

EA/TEF Child and Family Support Connection, Inc.
(Esophageal Artresia, Tracheoesophageal Fistula)
312-987-9085
www.eatef.org

Food Allergy and Anaphylaxis Network
800-929-4040
faan@foodallergy.org
www.foodallergy.org

Human Milk Banking Association of North America
919-787-5181
www.hmbana.org

La Leche League International
847-519-7730
www.lalecheleague.org
Breastfeeding the Baby with Reflux Booklet available from Le Leche
League International and PAGER Association

Mothers Overcoming Breastfeeding Issues
support@mobimotherhood.org
www.mobimotherhood.org

Kids with Food Allergies
215-230-5394
www.kidswithfoodallergies.org

Kids with Tubes (feeding)
Kidswithtubes.org
info@kidswithtubes.org

National Organization for Rare Disorders
203-744-0100
800-999-6673
orphan@rarediseases.org

Oley Foundation (Tube Feeding Support)
Albany Medical Center
800-776-OLEY
518-262-5079
www.oley.org

Pediatric Adolescent Gastroesophageal Reflux Association
P.O. Box 486
Buckeystown, Maryland 21717
301-601-9541
www.reflux.org
gergroup@aol.com

Professional Organizations

American Academy of Allergy, Asthma & Immunology
414-272-6071
Patient Information and Physician Referral Line: (800) 822-2762
info@aaaai.org

American Academy of Pediatrics
847-228-5005
www.aap.org
kidsdocs@aap.org

American College of Allergy, Asthma & Immunology
www.acaai.org
Mail@acaai.org

American College of Gastroenterology

703-820-7400
www.acg.org

American Gastroenterological Association
301-654-2055
www.gastro.org

National Digestive Disease Information Clearinghouse
National Institutes of Health
800-891-5389
www.digestive.niddk.nih.gov
nddic@info.niddk.nih.gov
www.niddk.nih.gov

North American Society for Pediatric Gastroenterology, Hepatology,
And Nutrition, NASPGHAN
215-233-0808

Travel Assistance for Medical Care

Angel Flight
888-4-AN-ANGEL
info@angelflight.org

National Association of Hospital Hospitality Houses, Inc.
NAHHH Inc.
800-542-9730
www.nahhh.org

PatientTravel.org
c/o Mercy Medical Airlift
757-318-9174
800-296-1217
www.mercymedical.org

Insurance Assistance

First Hand Foundation
816-201-1569
www.firsthandfoundation.org

Patient Advocate Foundation
800-532-5274
help@patientadvocate.org

A Consumer Guide to Handling Disputes with Your Employer or Private Health Plan, 2005 Update
http://www.consumersunion.org/health/hmo-review/

State Insurance Programs for Children
http://www.insurekidsnow.gov

Each state has a health insurance department. They should each have an ombudsman and a complaint line.

Family/Caregiver Support

National Family Caregivers Association
301-942-6430
www.nfcacares.org

Starbright Foundation
310-479-1212
800-315-2580
www.starbright.org

Genetic Research

Center for Genomic Sciences, Allegheny General Hospital, Pittsburgh
Inherited Pediatric GERD Study
888-887-7729
412-359-4707

MEET THE AUTHOR

I have worked in the non-profit arena for medical, environmental and consumer groups. I had my first exposure to the world of reflux when Katie was only twelve hours old and choked. Later, it became obvious that my son, Chris, had significant issues with reflux as a baby but was not diagnosed until much later. Eric and I had reflux as babies.

In 1992, I started a small support group as a way of getting help dealing with all the night waking, food refusal and constant crying. That small support group has taken on a life of its own and fourteen years later I am still the Executive Director of the Pediatric Adolescent Gastroesophageal Reflux Association. I am the author of three medical journals (Practical Gastroenterology, Neonatal Network, Zero to Three) and a contributing author on another (JAMA). I am the content administrator for www.reflux.org and the editor of Reflux Digest. I frequently speak to groups of early intervention workers, speech therapists and nurses.

I live in Garrett Park, MD. Write to me at Author@refluxbook.com.

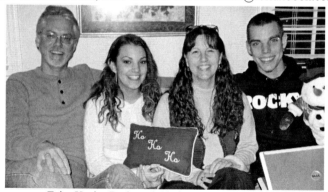

Eric, Katie, Beth and Chris – Christmas 2007

Child's Name

Date

Current Weight

Medication	Amount & details	Cross off times as you give the medicine					
Ranitidine	3cc - 30 min before meal	6am 10am 2pm 6pm 10pm					

Appendix A - Medication Chart (C) The Reflux Book

This table is also available on www.refluxbook.com
If you create a better table, send it and I can upload it.

Child's Name

Date

Symptoms	Amount & level	Timing or pattern comments	Total time	Grade
Crying	8 am—40 min shriek noon—45 min shriek 7-10 pm—fussy or crying	Started 30 min after bottle 30 min after bottle ??? No clue	4.5 hours	B-

Comments, questions, theories:

Appendix B - Symptoms Chart (C) The Reflux Book

This table is also available on www.refluxbook.com

Child's Name   Date   Current Weight   Age

In	Out	Diapers	Observations	Net Intake
3 oz carrots	1 oz carrots	wet	Threw up immediately. Overate?	+ 1 oz carrots

Copyright The Reflux Book 2007

Appendix C - Intake and Output Chart (C) The Reflux Book

This table is also available on www.refluxbook.com

INDEX

Before you check the Index, please check the Table of Contents